AF588168

PRAISE FOR *MY CHILD HAS AN EATING DISORDER*

"As a therapist who specializes in eating disorders, I wish every parent had this guide. I can't recommend it enough. Grateful to Jenny and Alli for providing a much-needed manual for families struggling with this painful disease."

—**Jenn Mann**, therapist, parenting expert, award-winning columnist, and author of *The A to Z Guide to Raising Happy, Confident Kids*

"Parenting a child with an eating disorder can be traumatic, because the stakes feel high and uncertainty can keep a family's nervous system in a constant state of alarm. *My Child Has an Eating Disorder* provides what stressed parents need most: clear, trustworthy information and a compassionate, trauma-informed roadmap that turns panic into a plan. It offers a compass and a map through perilous waters—steady, practical support that helps parents move toward safer ground and more effective action."

—**Robyn Koslowitz**, PhD, child psychologist, trauma specialist, and author of *Post-Traumatic Parenting: Break the Cycle and Become the Parent You Always Wanted to Be*

"For parents trying to make sense of eating disorders, this book is an essential starting point. It replaces fear and misinformation with knowledge and perspective."

—**Mark Steines**, Emmy-winning TV host

"Alli and Jenny have created a true gem for caregivers, clinicians, and anyone affected by eating disorders. Their Q&A format makes complex information clear, compassionate, and easy to navigate. For parents supporting a loved one, this book offers not just guidance but genuine comfort and hope."

—**Charlotte H. Markey,** PhD, professor of psychology at Rutgers University and author of *The Body Image Book* series

"As someone who struggled with an eating disorder as a child and into adulthood, I wish my mother and I had access to a thoughtful and informative book like *My Child Has an Eating Disorder* when I was a young girl."

—**Rebecca Morrison**, author of *The Blue Dress*

"A friendly orientation guide for parents researching the treatment landscape. It's so valuable to have clear direction from the start and this book puts that guidance right at your fingertips."

—**Eva Musby**, author of *Anorexia and Other Eating Disorders: How to Help Your Child Eat Well and Be Well*

"This! This is the book that has been needed for as long as eating disorders have been in existence. *My Child Has an Eating Disorder* is unlike any other resource to date. Alli and Jenny took mountains of research, practical lived experiences, and expert input, and they created a book that is a formidable resource yet approachable and very readable. *My Child Has an Eating Disorder* answers the myriad of questions that parents and loved ones have been desperately seeking answers to—I can hardly wait to share this book over and again."

—**Kathleen MacDonald**, former policy and communications director of the Eating Disorders Coalition and founder of Hope for Healing: The College Speaking Tour on Eating & Body Image Disorders

My Child Has an Eating Disorder

An Essential Guide for Parents of Kids, Teens, and Adults

Alli Spotts-De Lazzer, LMFT, CEDS-C

Jenny Mullaney, CCIEDC

BLOOMSBURY ACADEMIC
LONDON • NEW YORK • OXFORD • NEW DELHI • SYDNEY

BLOOMSBURY ACADEMIC
Bloomsbury Publishing Inc, 1359 Broadway, New York, NY 10018, USA
Bloomsbury Publishing Plc, 50 Bedford Square, London, WC1B 3DP, UK
Bloomsbury Publishing Ireland, 29 Earlsfort Terrace, Dublin 2, D02 AY28, Ireland

BLOOMSBURY, BLOOMSBURY ACADEMIC and the Diana logo are trademarks of Bloomsbury Publishing Plc

First published in the United States of America 2026

Library of Congress Cataloging-in-Publication Data
Names: Spotts-De Lazzer, Alli author | Mullaney, Jenny author
Title: My child has an eating disorder : an essential guide for parents of kids, teens, and adults / Alli Spotts-De Lazzer, LMFT, CEDS-C and Jenny Mullaney, CCIEDC.
Description: New York : Bloomsbury Academic, 2026. | Includes bibliographical references and index.
Identifiers: LCCN 2025053297 (print) | LCCN 2025053298 (ebook) |
ISBN 9798216377030 hb | ISBN 9798216377054 epdf | ISBN 9798216377047 ebook
Subjects: LCSH: Eating disorders in children | Eating disorders in adolescence
Classification: LCC RJ506.E18 S685 2026 (print) | LCC RJ506.E18 (ebook)
LC record available at https://lccn.loc.gov/2025053297
LC ebook record available at https://lccn.loc.gov/2025053298

ISBN: HB: 979-8-216-37703-0
ePDF: 979-8-216-37705-4
eBook: 979-8-216-37704-7

Typeset by Deanta Global Publishing Services, Chennai, India
Printed and bound in the United States of America

For product safety related questions contact productsafety@bloomsbury.com.

To find out more about our authors and books visit www.bloomsbury.com and sign up for our newsletters.

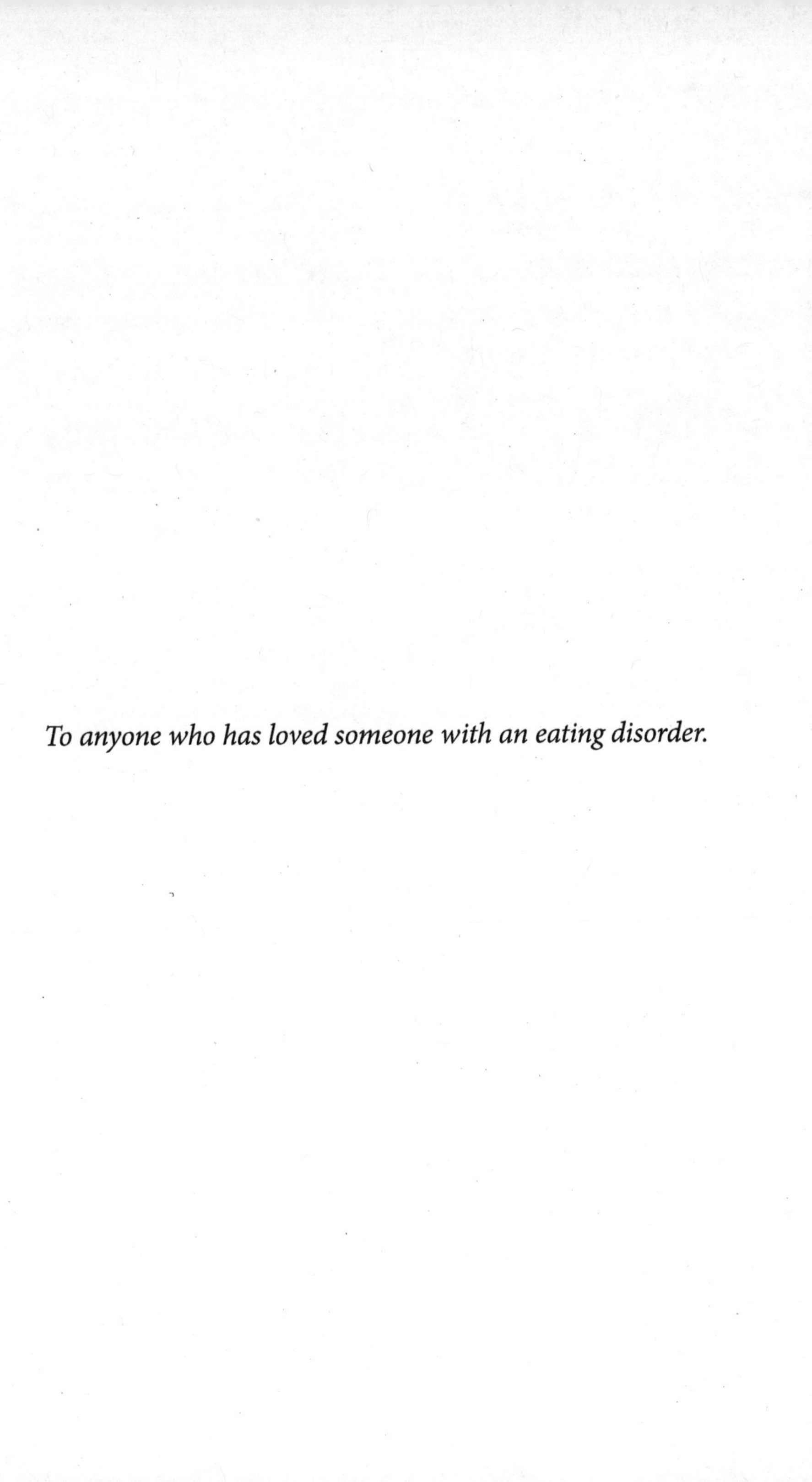

To anyone who has loved someone with an eating disorder.

Contents

Author's Note

Welcome! Before we begin, here's a short but important legal note.

My Child Has an Eating Disorder is intended for informational and educational purposes only and is not a substitute for professional medical, psychological, or nutritional advice, diagnosis, or treatment. Eating disorders are serious, complex illnesses, and advice from a qualified healthcare professional should be sought before making treatment decisions about medical and mental health concerns.

Alli Spotts-De Lazzer is a licensed mental health therapist and educator; Jenny Mullaney is a certified eating disorder recovery coach. Their collaboration reflects the inclusion of clinical treatment and non clinical support, offering readers insight from two distinct professional perspectives that are thoughtfully interwoven throughout this book. Reading these pages does not establish any professional relationship between the reader and the author(s).

Although the authors and publisher have made every effort to ensure that the information in this book was correct at the time of publication, the author and publisher do not assume and hereby disclaim any liability to any party for any loss, damage, or disruption caused by errors or omissions, whether such errors or omissions result from negligence, accident, or any other cause. Accordingly, neither the authors nor their publisher shall be liable for any direct, indirect, or consequential damages of any kind. Please note that resources mentioned (e.g., organizations and webpages) could change or become unavailable as time passes.

To protect privacy, where necessary, details have been altered, and some identifying information has been changed or combined; the heart of the examples and stories remains intact. Any trademarks, service marks, or copyrights mentioned are the property of their respective owners and do not indicate any relationship with the authors or publisher. Unless explicitly stated, any names of people, organizations, entities, or companies mentioned in these pages do not indicate any sponsorship or endorsement.

Please be aware before proceeding: This publication is about eating disorders, a sensitive topic. Though the authors and publisher have handled the content with consideration and care, portions of this book may feel upsetting to read. Additionally, health information may evolve and change over time. If at any time professional help is needed, reach out to a qualified medical or mental health provider.

Foreword

It is painful for any parent whenever their child has an illness. But when the illness is mysterious, with no blood tests available, and the child willfully engages in the symptoms and resists attempts by others to help them recover from it, it is excruciating. An eating disorder is such an illness. Eating disorders, like substance use disorders, have a behavioral component. In this kind of illness, the person engages in behaviors—for example, excessive drinking, or binging and purging—that lead to all sorts of unhealthy and life-interfering problems. With an alcohol problem, the person can abstain from drinking altogether. With an eating disorder, it's different; you cannot abstain from food; rather, you must learn how to regain a healthy relationship with food and your body. Healing from an eating disorder is very nuanced. Eating disorders are complex and multifactorial. There are biological, psychological, and cultural issues at play. There are treatments that are more likely to work than others, but no one treatment works for everyone. Each human with an eating disorder is different, and the jigsaw puzzle that led to each person's eating disorder is made up of very different pieces. Where does a parent go for help? There are websites, books, treatment centers, and organizations with varying information, so what's a parent to do? In 1996, I wrote the first edition of *Your Dieting Daughter* to help answer that question and revised it in 2006 because there was so much new information to share. Alli

Spotts-De Lazzer and Jenny Mullaney have now taken this task to a whole new level in their new book, *My Child Has an Eating Disorder: An Essential Guide for Parents of Kids, Teens, and Adults.* This book is truly a resource covering everything from definitions and terms to doctors' appointments, various treatment options, the new support service of eating disorder coaching, and much more. This combo team of therapist and coach, both recovered from their own eating disorders and both with years of expertise helping others recover, answer frequently asked questions and guide parents to the most updated resources. The book cannot tell any parent what to do, but the authors have collected and cut down to size volumes of material so that parents can have easy access to the most critical information and options to choose from. This is a book that can help many parents get started on the long path to help their child recover.

Carolyn Costin
The Carolyn Costin Institute
Author: *8 Keys to Recovery from an Eating Disorder*

Acknowledgments

Thank you to those who gave us their trust and time. We reached out to authorities on eating disorders and asked if they'd be willing to share their expertise with parents. They simply said *yes* and were generous. We are also grateful to each test reader who provided feedback on the original drafts of this book. Their diverse views challenged us to either revise, defend, clarify, or expand this guide's contents.

Each person's unique contributions and knowledge bases are part of why we believe this book will reach and help *many*. We stand behind the notion that when collective experiences and knowledge combine, the most thorough, thoughtful, and widely applicable resource possible can be created. (Seriously, this field has some truly brilliant minds with huge hearts.)

In alphabetical order, our expert contributors were:

- Carolyn Costin, MA, MEd, MFT, FAED, CEDS
- Vikas Duvvuri, MD, PhD
- Jenn Friedman, MA, LMHC
- Jennifer L. Gaudiani, MD, CEDS-C, FAED
- Rachel Goldstein, MD
- Jess Hudgens, MA, LPC, LCMHC, ASDCS, NCC

- Leslie Kaplan, MD, CEDS
- Michael Lutter, MD, PhD
- Charlotte Markey, PhD
- Lauren Muhlheim, PsyD, FAED, CEDS-C
- Rachel Presskreischer, PhD, MS
- Elyse Resch, MS, RDN, CEDRD-S, Fiaedp, FADA, FAND
- Chelsea Roff, C-IAYT

Many test and peer readers from a wide range of backgrounds provided feedback (in alphabetical order):

- Roxanne Acree, a Los Angeles-based writer, content creator, and comedian.
- Tammy Bagadassarian, the co-founder and executive director of Keystone Treatment, a mental health center providing evidence-based treatment for those struggling with eating disorders and mental health; a facilitator trainer for "The Body Project"; and a founding member of the Los Angeles Eating Disorder Collective.
- Jilly Becerra, a licensed marriage and family therapist, art therapist, clinical supervisor, and founder of Becerra Family Therapy, a psychotherapy group practice in Southern California that was founded on the vision of both training and providing bicultural and multilingual therapists and providers who are well-versed with LGBTQIA+ needs.
- Lisa Burns, a co-founder of International Eating Disorder Family Support and a past board and executive committee member of Families Empowered and Supporting Treatment of Eating Disorders (FEAST).

- Theresa Chesnut, a licensed clinical social worker and certified eating disorders specialist with over thirty years of experience, a trained internal family systems therapist, founder of the annual Tri-State Eating Disorder Conference, and owner and clinical director of The Chesnut Group with practices in California and Indiana.
- Heidi J. Dalzell, PsyD, a psychologist specializing in eating disorders, trauma, and psychedelic-assisted therapy with practices in New Jersey and Arizona; co-author of *A Clinician's Guide to Gender Identity and Body Image*, and author of *Eating Disorders and Body Image at Midlife: A Clinician's Guide.*
- Sue Detisch, the San Diego–based author of *Rest Now, Beloved*; a literature teacher; and a mother, grandmother, and devoted fur-mama.
- Steven Dunn, a Dallas-based attorney, founder of The Morgan Foundation, and activist in the eating disorder community.
- Karen Emmerman, PhD, an independent scholar of ecofeminist animal ethics, an affiliated instructor in the Department of Philosophy at the University of Washington, the education director of the Philosophy Learning and Teaching Organization, and an advisory board member of Food Empowerment Project.
- Winter Groeschl, a licensed professional counselor-supervisor, queer eating disorder clinician, dog mama, and grateful recovering eating disorder survivor.
- Olga Myszko, a board-certified pediatrician and adolescent medicine specialist at Tribeca Adolescent & Young Adult Medicine, the only concierge medicine practice in New York City that serves this population.

- Kevin Olmsted, the author of *Scared Dad Feeding*, a long-time member and current co-host of Men of FEAST, and the maker of the best slow-cooked chicken, steak sous vide, and shakshuka Jenny has ever tasted.
- Kristine Sinner, MS, a registered and licensed dietitian nutritionist, certified eating disorders specialist-consultant, the owner of Sinnergy Wellness Group, author of *Meal Planning Strategies, Tips, & Techniques: A Practical Handbook for Everyone*, and a medical nutrition therapist who has treated eating disorders since the early 1990s.
- Joy Zelikovsky, PsyD, MSCP, MA, MPhil Ed, MS Ed, a certified eating disorders specialist-consultant and the owner and director of Nourish the Heart Counseling and Growth Accelerated Therapy.

Of special note: Carolyn Costin, Jess Hudgens, Rachel Presskreischer, and Elyse Resch, thank you for going *above and beyond* in your contributions as experts *and* manuscript reviewers, too. Your generosity is abundant.

To the incredible community that helped make this possible—from answering quick questions, to providing legal consultation, to everything in between—Robyn Caruso, Barbara De Santis, Marise Freitas, Robin Gatter, Alexandra Halicki, Howard Kaufman, Michelle Massi, Ellen Morgan, Cindy Mullaney, Robert Nickel, Sara (Detisch) Peck, Dena Waxman, and William Hornby—you helped us during our most challenging moments! We appreciate you.

Louis Propp, PsyD, thank you for your kindness and time. Who knew our introduction would lead to Bloomsbury? Rachel Presskreischer, grateful to you for connecting us.

From Alli: To Michael De Lazzer, thank you for your enduring love, patience, and steady encouragement throughout this many-year journey. To Jenny, thank you for bringing your heartfelt perspective to the pages. Claudia Cagan—with gratitude.

To Jenny's friends, family, colleagues, and recovery coaching clients who supported, celebrated, and contributed to this endeavor, she is eternally grateful. A special thanks to Alli for her mentorship and belief in Jenny as a writer and coauthor. To Seven, you are the best road-cat a girl could have. And Carolyn, your unwavering love, guidance, and support have forever changed the course of Jenny's life and livelihood.

Bloomsbury and our managing editor, Christen Karniski, thank you for "getting it" and making sure this resource reaches the parents and caregivers who can benefit from it!

We appreciate each of your hearts, kindness, and generosity more than we can put into words . . .

Introduction

My Child Has an Eating Disorder: An Essential Guide for Parents of Kids, Teens, and Adults provides critical resources and tools to help parents navigate the crisis of an eating disorder. The authors, Alli Spotts-De Lazzer and Jenny Mullaney, draw from years of professional experience in the challenging field of eating disorders and from their personal journeys of recovery, offering insiders' tips to empower healing.

Alli Spotts-De Lazzer is a licensed marriage and family therapist, licensed professional clinical counselor, and certified eating disorders specialist recognized for her work with parents and her significant contributions to professional education in the eating disorders and mental health fields. She has published over one hundred trade and academic articles, created curriculum for the national certified eating disorders specialist credential, authored books, and lectured at major conferences. Jenny Mullaney is a certified eating disorder recovery coach widely respected for her specialty of live-in coaching. Her voice in this book offers a unique and previously unheard perspective—that of a trained provider who is immersed in the daily lives (twenty-four hours a day, seven days a week) of those who are healing, and their families.

Eating disorders can be confusing and overwhelming to experience. They are serious illnesses with significant medical and psychiatric consequences, and their high mortality rates are typically associated with suicide and medical complications.[1] If that frightens you, you've come to the right place.

Together, Alli and Jenny, "*we*," answer the crucial, pressing questions that parents and caregivers ask, arming you with the knowledge, wisdom, and resolve you will need as you walk this journey with your loved one. In these pages, you'll acquire information and a sense of direction that could otherwise take months or even years.

In creating this guide, we utilized relevant research, interviewed other experts, and took to heart the feedback of early test and peer-review readers with diverse backgrounds and knowledge of eating disorders. We also included direct quotes from other parents, caregivers, and clients who have been through eating disorders themselves. We provide well-rounded, practical information that touches on some of the many views and approaches you'll encounter as you expand your knowledge of eating disorders—all centralized in one place for your convenience.

My Child Has an Eating Disorder can aid anyone in a parent or caregiver role whose kid, teen, or adult

- has been recently diagnosed with an eating disorder, such as anorexia nervosa, avoidant/restrictive food intake disorder (ARFID), binge-eating disorder, bulimia nervosa, or other specified/unspecified feeding or eating disorder (OSFED/UFED), and is considering treatment
- is underway in the treatment process
- has tried seemingly *everything* without significant success.

Please note that this book may also be helpful for parents and caregivers who believe their loved one *might* have an eating disorder or related concern.

In an accessible Q and A format, these pages can be read sequentially or as topics become relevant. Each chapter is devoted to a major area of concern that parents and caregivers face when supporting their loved one with an eating disorder.

- Chapter 1, "Initial Questions," equips you with the necessary foundational knowledge of eating disorders.
- Chapter 2, "Empathy and Understanding," allows you to better comprehend what your loved one might be experiencing.
- Chapter 3, "Cultural Myths and Messages," explores societal misconceptions about eating disorders and diet culture.
- Chapter 4, "Preparing for Treatment," assists you in navigating treatment decisions and options.
- Chapter 5, "About Treatment," prepares you for life during treatment.
- Chapter 6, "Obstacles to Healing," helps you overcome common hurdles that can impede your loved one's recovery.
- Chapter 7, "Hope and Help," gives voice to those with personal experience of eating disorders, adding firsthand lessons and hindsight.

As you read, please take note of what *you* feel could benefit you and your loved one. Notice when you hear your brain say, "I agree with that" or "Huh? I haven't thought of that before." Sometimes, what we share may need to be modified or individualized to better meet the specific needs of your child and family.

Origin

After years of working with parents of kids, teens, and adults with eating disorders, Alli noticed that caregivers asked the same questions repeatedly. As if eating disorders aren't challenging enough with all the misinformation out there, the resources, although comprehensive, seemed spread out, and parents didn't know where to turn. The idea for this book was born.

We had just finished working together on a case where we experienced the power of a recovery coach paired with a strong clinical lead within a collaborative treatment team. Our distinct yet complementary backgrounds—one grounded in treatment and the other in hands-on support—held meaningful potential. What could happen if we combined forces?

So Alli shared the concept for this book with Jenny. As it turned out, we had both been receiving many of the *same* repeat inquiries from parents, which made our mutual calling obvious: We developed this essential guide to provide clear answers and support. It's awful to feel lost, scared, and confused about where and how to begin. We wrote this book to help.

Combined, Alli and Jenny have dedicated decades to helping people with eating disorders and their families break free from these illnesses. Our hope is that the thoughts, tools, exercises, and candidness contained in this book will help you and your relationship with your loved one who has the eating disorder.

Background

There are many perspectives and beliefs about healing eating disorders, which can get confusing as you gather information. We share our backgrounds and clarify our roles to provide the context behind our views and approaches.

We are both strongly influenced by the philosophies and teachings of Carolyn Costin, a pioneer in the field of eating disorders and an internationally recognized expert. Costin founded the first residential treatment center for eating disorders in a home-like setting. A pillar of her work is that full recovery (*recovered*, past tense) is possible. Most recently, she established the Carolyn Costin Institute (CCI), which trains and certifies eating disorder recovery coaches. While the certification is not state- or nationally regulated, it has become well-known and respected by many within the eating disorders field.

Jenny's work as a recovery coach has been overseen by Costin since 2017. She describes the process of becoming a CCI coach as rigorous. It includes a multi-module course and an extensive supervised internship with continuing education.

As a recovery coach, Jenny helps her clients in real time with tasks they may find overwhelming after stepping outside their therapist's or dietitian's office. She leaves the clinical psychological work to the therapist, the nutritional guidance to the dietitian, and the medical oversight to the doctor, but collaborates with them to echo, reinforce, and execute their messaging. Her approach to this work is relationship-focused and tailored to each individual.

Jenny is one of the few recovery coaches who *lives with* clients and their families. During a stay in someone's home, she can offer an outsider's perspective while getting an insider's view. When working collaboratively with the other practitioners, Jenny's support as a live-in recovery coach has been able to help the treatment team to crack the code of what is keeping a client, along with their family, trapped in a revolving door of treatment, discharge, relapse, repeat.

Alli began her clinical work in 2007. Her foundation was shaped by early training at a residential treatment facility under Costin and a community agency where she developed a small eating disorders outpatient program, followed by a few years of consultation in Costin-led groups. Since then, Alli expanded her training to incorporate a wide range of therapeutic approaches for eating disorders, including evidence-based (methodically scientifically tested), evidence-informed (based on or influenced by research findings), and trauma-informed (incorporating the influence of trauma in treatment). Her eclectic approach allows her to draw from multiple frameworks guided by what resonates with and empowers each client's healing.

Alli is a licensed therapist and certified eating disorders specialist; each designation requires specific education along with thousands of hours of training and practice. As such, she develops comprehensive treatment plans (individualized roadmaps for healing) and often brings in other team members needed to meet the standard of care, such as a dietitian, psychiatrist, and medical doctor. In her role as an eating disorders therapist, Alli provides therapy that usually includes exploring misleading, unhelpful thoughts and behaviors and guiding the person toward more accurate, helpful ones. She offers psychoeducation, which means arming clients and families with eating disorders education, research, and information. Through this therapeutic work, clients learn about their emotions, address what could be contributing to or sustaining their eating disorder, and more. The process helps individuals to identify strategies that support recovery-oriented change while addressing other potential psychiatric diagnoses, working through the effects of trauma, and improving relationship dynamics with self and others.

The two of us have complementary philosophies about healing. Similar to how we take a team approach in treatment settings, we collaborated to create these pages. Though we are distinct in our roles as therapist and recovery coach, we understand how to support our mutual clients, their families, and each other in harmony. Our writing reflects that.

Terminology

In this book, the terms *kid*, *kiddo*, *child*, and *your loved one* are synonymous and can apply to an adult or minor. People of any age can be afflicted with eating disorders. Additionally, eating disorders can leave a person stuck developmentally, meaning younger than their actual age in various ways (emotionally, hormonally, behaviorally, etc.).

When we say *parent* or *caregiver*, we're referencing people who are responsible for overseeing someone else's well-being. That includes guardians, grandparents, siblings, extended family, friends, chosen family, and more. We use parent and caregiver interchangeably.

Providers frequently use the terms *client* and *patient* interchangeably. For consistency and ease of reading, this book mostly uses *client*.

Throughout, we'll refer to the team member who covers the nutrition therapy aspect of eating disorders treatment as a *dietitian*. We do this to prevent confusion. The *nutritionist* title may be affiliated with formal training and regulated healthcare, such as the certified nutrition specialist (CNS). However, in some areas, anyone is allowed to call themselves a nutritionist, even someone with *no* background or education in nutrition. On a similar note, many types of therapists exist. Unless otherwise specified, in these pages, the term denotes a licensed, regulated mental health therapist or counselor.

Regulated professionals (e.g., doctors, dietitians, and licensed therapists) have state or national policies that set educational and training requirements as well as boards that oversee ethics, conduct, and compliance. In the United States, most *clinical* providers are regulated; *clinical* means direct care, such as assessment, diagnosis, and treatment. In this context, *nonclinical* indicates supportive care, such as the work of recovery coaches.

Finally, in mental health and eating disorder recovery spaces, we strive to emphasize a person-first language (e.g., person with bulimia, person who binges) instead of labels (e.g., bulimic, binger). We believe that people are more than their diagnoses.

Setting the Stage

We're both based in the United States. Especially if you're in another country and reading this, we invite you to adapt concepts to your healthcare systems.

Eating disorders are expensive to treat. That's partially because they involve psychological, nutritional, and medical domains. Usually, a single provider is not trained and licensed in all three. So, it can require three different providers and their fees. Further, insurance can be tricky about coverage for these disorders. Much of what we offer in this book would be optimal if you have the resources (e.g., time, money, and specialized providers). And then there's reality: People often must find ways to achieve their treatment goals with limited funds and a lack of access to the ideal treatment providers. We've done our best to address both.

There are many philosophies about treating eating disorders, how people heal, etc. Even with the well-researched approaches that offer guidance and structure, a lot can be left to figure out during the healing journey. So, take a deep exhale and please say this to yourself: "It's OK to not know what to do right now; I'll take this step by step." This book can be your guide to breaking down the crisis of an eating disorder into manageable parts.

Finally, although it's changing in current times, for the most part, older eating disorders research was conducted in homogenized subject pools, such as affluent, young, white females.[2] Thus, science has produced mainly treatment options derived from their effectiveness in this group. However, eating disorders affect all races, cultures, genders, ethnicities, socioeconomic statuses, ages, sexual orientations, marginalized populations, sizes, etc. You get the picture. So please keep in mind when we—or others, for that matter—refer to research, that could be the case.

Expectations

This book is a unique, behind-the-scenes experience rather than information that is easily at one's fingertips online. We offer quick-to-read, real-life answers that often include referrals to additional reading and resources. In these pages, we've identified various learning outlets, options, and portals to more in-depth information.

We need to be clear, though. We cannot provide treatment or teach you how to treat eating disorders here—that usually takes thousands of hours of formal training and a professional license.[3]

Most importantly, in the painful moments, these pages will provide you with a sense of community and hope. We've healed. We've witnessed people who have healed. And we've seen families that have healed. We strongly believe a home environment that supports recovery can make a positive difference during this process. You are already making choices to support your loved one's ongoing healing by picking up this book.

Though no book can tell you *exactly* what to do, by the last page, when you add together the questions and answers that apply to you and your situation, we believe that you'll be better equipped to decide what to do when your child has an eating disorder.

You're here, and that matters. Let's begin.

1

Initial Questions

We recognize how overwhelmed a parent may feel when their kid, teen, or adult child has an eating disorder. This chapter covers foundational information that can be helpful—even necessary—for supporting a loved one of any age.

What's the first thing I should do if my loved one has an eating disorder?

Exactly what you are doing right now: *learning* about eating disorders. Though celebrities, social media, and the COVID-19 pandemic have created more public awareness of eating disorders, they can still seem confusing and frightening, from historical misconceptions about them to physical complications caused by them. With time, physical risks are likely to increase, and the eating disorder beliefs and behaviors can become more ingrained. Research shows that early intervention is key.[1] Understandably, you may feel a sense of urgency. It can be a balancing act between moving swiftly and having enough information to make thoughtful decisions.

Especially if eating disorders are brand new to you, the following will likely benefit you to understand immediately: the *Nine Truths About Eating Disorders* along with the complexities and physical complications of eating disorders. We unpack each below.

Nine Truths About Eating Disorders

Dispelling nine of the most common, long-standing myths about eating disorders, we find the document the *Nine Truths* to be the most in-a-nutshell version of what you need to know.[2] The Academy for Eating Disorders spearheaded the creation of the *Nine Truths,* and Alli was co-chair of the committee that brought the project to fruition at the time. At this point, the content has been endorsed by more than thirty eating disorders organizations. That's a rare level of consensus in the field, which we believe can give parents confidence in the points.

As you read, notice if you find yourself agreeing, feeling relieved, disagreeing, or finding yourself surprised. You can rest assured that science does back these statements.[3]

1. Many people with eating disorders look healthy yet may be extremely ill.
2. Families are not to blame and can be the patients' and providers' best allies in treatment.
3. An eating disorder diagnosis is a health crisis that disrupts personal and family functioning.
4. Eating disorders are not choices, but serious biologically influenced illnesses.
5. Eating disorders affect people of all genders, ages, races, ethnicities, body shapes and weights, sexual orientations, and socioeconomic statuses.

6. Eating disorders carry an increased risk for both suicide and medical complications.
7. Genes and environment play important roles in the development of eating disorders.
8. Genes alone do not predict who will develop eating disorders.
9. Full recovery from an eating disorder is possible. Early detection and intervention are important.

Awareness of these *Nine Truths* could prevent potential blocks or interferences to the healing process.

Complexities and Physical Complications of Eating Disorders

Though eating disorders are officially classified as *mental* disorders, they are fairly unique in that they are inherently intertwined with nutritional and medical aspects. So we invite you to start getting used to a mindset shift: Consider what is not intuitive about a *mental* disorder—health, nutritional, and medical issues in addition to the psychological aspects.

It can be alarming to hear, but there are many physical risks. Eating disorders can affect nearly every system in the body.[4] Depending on which eating disorder, complications may include but are not limited to experiencing malnutrition, anemia, acid reflux, bloating, diarrhea/constipation, osteoporosis/osteopenia, arrhythmias, blood pressure issues, electrolyte imbalance, dehydration, multiple organ failure, and more.[5] Your anxiety might be spiking at this moment. You can probably see why the involvement of a medical professional is part of the standard of care for eating disorders.

If you'd like to learn more *right now* about the medical assessment and management of the eating disorder, please feel free to jump ahead in this chapter to the relevant Q and As. (See the **Should my child go to a doctor immediately?** and **What if the doctor gives my child a clean bill of health?** sections.) Note: For any issues that could be urgent, consider going to your nearest emergency room.

What are eating disorders?

Eating disorders are psychiatric illnesses that often result in physical or medical consequences, and their main marker is eating difficulties. This section may feel heavy on jargon. However, you will benefit from understanding the basics of the most common eating disorders before reading further. (That's so we all start off on the same page, literally and metaphorically speaking.)

For your understanding, below are brief, typical-ish snapshots of the diagnoses this book covers (in alphabetical order): anorexia nervosa, avoidant/restrictive food intake disorder, binge-eating disorder, bulimia nervosa, and other specified/unspecified feeding or eating disorder. Each is followed by the current criteria per the *Diagnostic and Statistical Manual of Mental Disorders, Fifth Edition, Text Revision* (*DSM-5-TR*). Later in this chapter, you'll find information on who can officially diagnose these conditions. (See the **How does my child get a diagnosis?** section).

Anorexia Nervosa

Snapshot: A person with anorexia nervosa refuses to eat or restricts intake, oftentimes to get thinner. They are usually terrified of gaining weight and can't see or assess their body accurately. The field now recognizes that people at any weight, shape, or size—not just the emaciated look that the media has traditionally shown—can develop this disorder, which is currently called atypical anorexia nervosa.

For a diagnosis of anorexia nervosa, each of the following criteria must be satisfied:[6]

A. Restriction of energy intake relative to requirements, leading to a significantly low body weight in the context of age, sex, developmental trajectory, and physical health. *Significantly low weight* is defined as a weight that is less than minimally normal or, for children and adolescents, less than that minimally expected.

B. Intense fear of gaining weight or of becoming fat, or persistent behavior that interferes with weight gain, even though at a significantly low weight.

C. Disturbance in the way in which one's body weight or shape is experienced, undue influence of body weight or shape on self-evaluation, or persistent lack of recognition of the seriousness of the current low body weight.

Did you notice all the *or* conjunctions? When paying attention to those, anorexia nervosa may not match the stereotypes we all are exposed to, such as when someone has anorexia nervosa and does *not* have an intense fear of gaining weight.

There are two subtypes of anorexia nervosa. The restricting subtype is when binge-purge episodes haven't regularly happened during the last three months, and the binge-eating/purging subtype is when they have.[7] Here, bingeing means feeling a loss of control while eating *a lot* in a certain amount of time. Purging means using methods to forcefully empty the body of food or calories in an attempt to control weight (e.g., self-induced vomiting, abusing laxatives or diuretics, or misusing insulin if a person has diabetes).[8]

Avoidant/Restrictive Food Intake Disorder

Snapshot: A person with avoidant/restrictive food intake disorder (ARFID) displays extreme food preferences beyond pickiness. There is often an aversion to many tastes, textures, or temperatures and a lack of hunger cues or interest in food. A fear of consequences from eating, such as choking or vomiting, may exist. All of these can show up as restrictive intake. This person can be any age, from a very young child to an elderly adult. Interestingly, research has been showing that autism and ARFID often co-occur.[9]

For a diagnosis of ARFID, each of the following criteria must be satisfied:[10]

- **A.** An eating or feeding disturbance (e.g., apparent lack of interest in eating or food; avoidance based on the sensory characteristics of food; concern about aversive consequences of eating) associated with one (or more) of the following:
  1. Significant weight loss (or failure to achieve expected weight gain or faltering growth in children).
  2. Significant nutritional deficiency.
  3. Dependence on enteral feeding or oral nutritional supplements.
  4. Marked interference with psychosocial functioning.
- **B.** The disturbance is not better explained by lack of available food or by an associated culturally sanctioned practice.
- **C.** The eating disturbance does not occur exclusively during the course of anorexia nervosa or bulimia nervosa, and there is no evidence of a disturbance in the way in which one's body weight or shape is experienced.

D. The eating disturbance is not attributable to a concurrent medical condition or not better explained by another mental disorder. When the eating disturbance occurs in the context of another condition or disorder, the severity of the eating disturbance exceeds that routinely associated with the condition or disorder and warrants additional clinical attention.

Binge-Eating Disorder

Snapshot: A person with binge-eating disorder regularly eats large quantities of food, feels out of control while doing it, and experiences tremendous guilt, sadness, or stress about it.

For a diagnosis of binge-eating disorder, each of the following criteria must be satisfied:[11]

A. Recurrent episodes of binge eating. An episode of binge eating is characterized by both of the following:

1. Eating, in a discrete period of time (e.g., within any 2-hour period), an amount of food that is definitely larger than most people would eat in a similar period of time under similar circumstances.
2. A sense of lack of control over eating during the episode (e.g., a feeling that one cannot stop eating or control what or how much one is eating).

B. The binge-eating episodes are associated with three (or more) of the following:

1. Eating much more rapidly than normal.
2. Eating until feeling uncomfortably full.
3. Eating large amounts of food when not feeling physically hungry.

4. Eating alone because of feeling embarrassed by how much one is eating.
5. Feeling disgusted with oneself, depressed, or very guilty afterward.

C. Marked distress regarding binge eating is present.

D. The binge eating occurs, on average, at least once a week for 3 months.

E. The binge eating is not associated with the recurrent use of inappropriate compensatory behavior as in bulimia nervosa and does not occur exclusively during the course of bulimia nervosa or anorexia nervosa.

Bulimia Nervosa

Snapshot: A person with bulimia nervosa regularly eats large quantities of food, feels out of control while doing it, and tries to compensate for the binges by vomiting, using laxatives, fasting, working out excessively, misusing insulin, or other methods. This person tends to judge themself as good or bad by their body size, shape, or weight.

For a diagnosis of bulimia nervosa, each of the following criteria must be satisfied:[12]

A. Recurrent episodes of binge eating. An episode of binge eating is characterized by both of the following:

1. Eating, in a discrete period of time (e.g., within any 2-hour period), an amount of food that is definitely larger than what most individuals would eat in a similar period of time under similar circumstances.
2. A sense of lack of control over eating during the episode (e.g., a feeling that one cannot stop eating or control what or how much one is eating).

B. Recurrent inappropriate compensatory behaviors in order to prevent weight gain, such as self-induced vomiting; misuse of laxatives, diuretics, or other medications; fasting; or excessive exercise.

C. The binge eating and inappropriate compensatory behaviors both occur, on average, at least once a week for 3 months.

D. Self-evaluation is unduly influenced by body shape and weight.

E. The disturbance does not occur exclusively during episodes of anorexia nervosa.

Other Specified/Unspecified Feeding or Eating Disorder

Snapshot: Other specified feeding or eating disorder (OSFED) and unspecified feeding or eating disorder (UFED) are your catchall categories for those whose behaviors and attitudes don't exactly match the criteria used to diagnose anorexia nervosa, ARFID, binge-eating disorder, or bulimia nervosa.

Per the *DSM-5-TR*, OSFED applies to the following: "Presentations in which symptoms characteristic of a feeding and eating disorder that cause clinically significant distress or impairment in social, occupational, or other important areas of functioning predominate but do not meet the full criteria for any of the disorders in the feeding and eating disorders diagnostic class."[13] Examples of OSFED include but are not limited to (in alphabetical order):[14]

- atypical anorexia nervosa, such as anorexia nervosa without low weight
- atypical binge-eating disorder, such as behaviors occur fewer than once a week

- atypical bulimia nervosa, such as behaviors occur fewer than once a week
- night eating syndrome, such as excessive eating at night (e.g., post-dinner and waking up to eat)
- purging disorder, such as regularly purging for weight control without bingeing.

And finally, UFED "includes presentations in which there is insufficient information to make a more specific diagnosis (e.g., in emergency room settings)."[15]

Those are the basics of the eating disorders this book covers, but a person may not stay at one diagnosis. Along the journey, one eating disorder diagnosis might change to another. For example,

- If someone with anorexia nervosa binge-purge subtype gains enough weight, their diagnosis often shifts to bulimia nervosa. Also, a substantial proportion of people with anorexia nervosa restrictive subtype eventually migrate to binge-purge behaviors or bulimia nervosa.[16]
- If someone with binge-eating disorder starts using compensatory behaviors (e.g., fasting most of the day or purging), their diagnosis may become bulimia nervosa.
- If someone with anorexia nervosa, binge-eating disorder, or bulimia nervosa no longer meets the full criteria for the diagnosis (e.g., due to less frequent behaviors), their diagnosis might change to OSFED—because they are getting well!

It gets complicated to list all the ways a diagnosis may change throughout the course of an illness. Diagnostic crossover (the fancy term) is mentioned here because if it happens, it can feel jolting or scary to a parent as well as the person with an eating disorder.

Understanding the basics of these disorders can help you manage what a crossover might mean for you and your loved one.

What if my child's food and body image issues don't match a specific diagnosis?

That can happen for so many reasons—from understandings of eating disorders continuing to evolve to people having symptoms that don't entirely match existing criteria, to eating disorders presenting differently among genders, to people with eating disorders being guarded or secretive about their behaviors. (That last one means that your child may be doing and thinking things in secret.) Be curious and compassionate about what is going on for them, as it may lead to a clearer understanding of *their* specific struggles.

The subsequent terms, as titled, are not currently formal diagnoses in the *Diagnostic and Statistical Manual of Mental Disorders, Fifth Edition, Text Revision* (*DSM-5-TR*) but may fall into the other specified feeding or eating disorder (OSFED) diagnosis. Or, they could be a component of a different diagnosis already described in this chapter. (See the **What are eating disorders?** section.) Each term deserves attention, and short descriptions are included so you can have them on your radar (in alphabetical order): bigorexia, chewing and spitting, compulsive exercise, diabulimia, orthorexia as well as orthorexia nervosa, and subjective bingeing.

Bigorexia

This refers to a seeming obsession with bulking up and musculature. This might look like the person fixating on muscles and size, going to the gym, protein powders, steroids, etc. Bigorexia is a preoccupation with increasing muscle mass and a form of muscle dysmorphia,[17] which is under the body dysmorphic disorders title in the *DSM-5-TR*. It often includes disordered eating. It can also happen as part of or alongside an eating disorder. There is a debate about whether bigorexia should be considered an eating disorder.[18]

Chewing and Spitting

This refers to chewing the taste out of food and spitting out the contents. It appeared in the *Diagnostic and Statistical Manual of Mental Disorders, Fourth Edition, Text Revision (DSM-IV-TR)*, but not in the *DSM-5*. Sometimes used as a compensatory behavior, chewing and spitting can occur across the range of eating disorders.[19]

Compulsive Exercise

This refers to a pattern of over exercising, often showing up as a person who exercises excessively or uses compulsive physical activity to "burn off" what they ate. When it comes to compulsive exercise, the person typically feels driven—they *must* be active according to their rules—and it may be an attempt to manage distress or avoid a feared consequence (e.g., If I don't do this, something bad will happen).[20] This may be a feature of various eating disorders.

Diabulimia

This refers to the combination of type 1 diabetes mellitus (T1DM) and insulin misuse as a form of weight control.[21] The person may appear to drop weight rapidly, have persistently high blood sugar levels, experience episodes of diabetic ketoacidosis (DKA), face hospitalizations due to treatment irregularity, and many more potential signs.[22] Important: Purging via limiting or omitting insulin is an extremely dangerous practice.

Orthorexia and Orthorexia Nervosa

Both refer to a rigid focus on eating only healthy or pure foods. Either might look like the person who prides themself on practicing "pure" or "clean" eating. In reality, they've lost their choice about what they eat. For example, maybe they go on vacation and can't eat much or any selections because foods don't feel pure or safe enough, and that scares them.

You may be wondering if there's a difference when the words are so often used interchangeably. Orthorexia nervosa is characterized by an extreme obsession with or fixation on healthy eating, and orthorexia (without the nervosa) is basically a less severe, less life-interrupting version.[23] As of now, there is no official diagnosis in the *DSM-5-TR*, but clinicians often view it as fitting within OSFED or anorexia nervosa without fear of weight gain.[24]

Subjective Bingeing

This refers to eating a small to seemingly "normal" amount of food but experiencing it as a binge. For example, we've worked with therapy and recovery coaching clients who have expressed torment over what they perceived as a binge. When asked what they ate, their answers may surprise you. One that still stands out to Alli came from early in her career: "two bites of a sandwich."

Particularly if you're in the United States, you may also want to familiarize yourself with the eating disorder diagnostic descriptions in the *International Classification of Diseases (ICD)*, which is maintained by the World Health Organization.[25] Why? Both the *ICD* and the *DSM* can be important not only for understanding codes on superbills (receipts for reimbursement) and insurance paperwork, but for creating a more complete picture.

Diagnosis coding for insurance in the United States is typically *ICD*-based while the *DSM* governs criteria. (If you find it confusing that they can differ from each other, we agree!) For instance, the *ICD 11* recognizes subjective binges in bulimia nervosa and binge-eating disorder. At the time of this writing, the most recent *DSM*—the *DSM-5-TR*—does not include subjective binges, but that could have changed by the time you're reading this. The American Psychiatric Association updates every few years, and the current version will be most accurate.[26] You can usually locate eating disorder diagnostic criteria online, at no cost, by using a straightforward internet search.

What *kind* of binges (subjectively or objectively large amounts of food) can be important to understand due to the potential psychological, nutritional, and medical consequences of the behavior. Subjective bingeing may also contribute to a misinterpretation of symptoms—for example, if someone reports binges that aren't objectively large amounts of food, they could be given a diagnosis that does not match their experience.

In conclusion, with all the nuances, delineating one diagnosis from another can feel challenging! And your child's symptoms might not fit a diagnosis as written. When in doubt, focus on the beliefs and behaviors. Hopefully, you'll have the opportunity to work with a trained, licensed, or appropriately credentialed professional who can best diagnose, track what's happening or changing, and assess the risks associated with behaviors. That can help tremendously and inform effective treatment.

How does my child get a diagnosis?

There are two parts to this question. First, in many states, medical doctors, physician assistants, nurse practitioners, and licensed mental health therapists can typically provide an eating disorder diagnosis per the most current *Diagnostic and Statistical Manual of Mental Disorders (DSM)* by the American Psychiatric Association—but not a dietitian or recovery coach. Second, for your and your child's awareness, a provider experienced in eating disorders, including many dietitians and some recovery coaches, may help you recognize whether thoughts and behaviors might seem consistent with an eating disorder. Frightened parents often reach out to whichever provider they find first so they have an idea of how to proceed.

Should my child go to a doctor immediately?

When something could be wrong medically, it's always a good idea to consult a physician (or other qualified medical provider, such as a nurse practitioner or physician assistant). Don't rely on "my child *looks* OK" to determine whether to see a doctor. We've known many people with eating disorders who *look* fine but are not medically stable.

A doctor can assess basic, current medical stability, and if necessary, provide a helpful specialist referral. If your child is a minor, talk to their pediatrician about your concerns; if your child is an adult, ask them to go to their primary care provider. You might inquire whether basic vitals (blood pressure, pulse, temperature, etc.) and blood work will be part of the visit. These are commonly included in medical evaluations for people with eating disorders and can help a doctor check if there are medical issues needing immediate attention.

Heads-up: If you cannot find a doctor already familiar with eating disorders, the Academy for Eating Disorders (AED) created the booklet *Eating Disorders: A Guide to Medical Care*, which is available online.[27] It provides specific laboratory work recommendations and vital information. You may want to send this booklet to your child's pediatrician before their appointment. Or if they're an adult, ask them to take it with them. And if they say no or that you're being ridiculous worrying, know that this happens.

There are times when a person with an eating disorder is not willing to get a medical evaluation. Perhaps they are an adult, and the parent has no authority or bargaining chips to get them to a physician. As a therapist, Alli has found herself in this familiar position (so she has empathy!). Here is a quick example from her work that might help you:

> A client would *not* acknowledge having an eating disorder, let alone ask a doctor to target relevant tests and assessments. But time was of the essence. Since the client was convinced the medical visit was unnecessary and the physician would agree, I encouraged them to tell their doctor that they thought their therapist was "overreacting" by worrying and suggesting a check-up—essentially, "Blame me!"
>
> That framing helped them feel comfortable enough to make the appointment and also to bring up my concerns about (1) potential malnutrition and effects of undereating and (2) the possible impact on their heart. They also agreed to ask the doctor to check for anything that could affect their moods or require them to limit their exercise practices.
>
> When I first did this, I remember immediately calling Leslie Kaplan, MD, certified eating disorders specialist (CEDS), located in Calabasas, California. I explained the whole situation.
>
> Dr. Kaplan confirmed that the framing I had used (e.g., undernutrition) could help a non-specialist doctor to better target appropriate medical assessments that matched this client's behaviors and risks. She added that having the doctor sign off on a medical evaluation as simple as "So-and-so is safe for weekly

outpatient therapy sessions without restrictions on exercise" could be a starting point to assess safety in the moment. She relayed that most doctors will, at the very least, check general and orthostatic vitals (a series of blood pressure and pulse measurements taken in different positions to assess how a patient responds to changes in posture) before signing that.[28]

It wasn't ideal, but it was *something*. And, as a result, my client was open to obtaining the assurance I needed.

The medical oversight piece can be challenging to achieve and monitor at times. Other caregivers have found a variety of ways to get their loved ones evaluated by a doctor. Just ask them for ideas. They'll probably be happy to share. We provide leads to caregiver-focused support groups later in this chapter. (See the **Why should I make attending a support group a priority?** and **How do I find a support group?** sections.)

Finally, because medical risks and complications can be a significant part of eating disorders, it's especially valuable to understand those pieces. In 2025, Dr. Jennifer Gaudiani published the second edition of her classic 2018 book, *Sick Enough: A Guide to the Medical Complications of Eating Disorders and Undernutrition*, a reader-friendly book for laypeople.[29] This book has been helpful to many parents, clinicians, and people with eating disorders. If you are not in a position to buy *Sick Enough*, check if your local library carries it. If they don't, please request that they do.

What if the doctor gives my child a clean bill of health?

You're probably breathing a sigh of relief! However, here is why that clean bill of health might be false reassurance.

Most doctors and other medical providers are not well-trained in eating disorders—if at all. A 2015 study in the United States showed us that of 637 residency programs, 514 (eighty percent) did not offer any eating disorder rotations.[30] Though there may have been improvements in recent years, a 2021 study showed how variable training can still be. Of 162 emergency room physicians, less than two percent of them had completed an eating disorders rotation during residency. The majority did not know about major eating disorders treatment guidelines or even a publication called *ED* (Emergency Department) *Management of Patients with Eating Disorders.*[31]

That is not to criticize doctors or other medical providers; it's to inform parents why those in healthcare might not perform the proper protocols for eating disorders or may provide false reassurance. We reached out to Rachel Goldstein, MD, a Clinical Associate Professor in Adolescent Medicine at Stanford Medicine Children's Health and an eating disorders expert, to say more about this conundrum. She shared the following:

> Medical signs and symptoms of eating disorders can be vague and sometimes overlap with other conditions. For example, when a young person loses their menstrual period, depending on their age, it may be chalked up to the normal variation that we can see—especially if that happens within the first two years after starting their period. However, losing a period in the setting of inadequate nutrition and weight loss is a very concerning sign that the body is shutting down systems to conserve energy. The main concern we have with losing periods, also known as amenorrhea, is the potential for negative effects on bone health during a critical time for bone growth. While fertility is often impaired with amenorrhea, it typically resolves with weight restoration.

I've seen patients who, before seeing me as an eating disorder expert, had seen an OB/GYN for their missing period or a cardiologist for a low heart rate. They (and their parents) were reassured without necessarily digging in further as to why the periods went away in the first place or why the heart rate was so low.

Another scenario I've seen often affects patients struggling with eating disorders at higher weights. These are the kids who were maybe counseled in the past to adopt healthy lifestyle changes. They decided to "be healthy" but ended up severely restricting their intake and losing weight way too quickly. These people (who may be more likely to be black and brown, given the disparities that we see in folks at higher weight) are often initially praised for their weight loss. The people surrounding them usually don't realize how they went about the weight loss or that they have now developed an eating disorder.

Also, there is still a lot of bias around "who gets an eating disorder." Think young, Caucasian, and female. So, people who struggle with eating disorders but don't fit the mold can be missed and deemed healthy without a closer look.

The common thread in these scenarios is this: Medical providers didn't take a step back to look at the bigger picture and context for the symptoms that they were seeing. Sometimes this happens because our healthcare system isn't set up to give the time needed during visits to have these conversations. Sometimes providers may not be well-trained in eating disorders, which may lead them to evaluate a symptom in isolation and miss the bigger context.

What can a parent do? Dr. Goldstein provides suggestions for dealing with healthcare providers when seeking help for their loved ones:

1. The best advice I have is to be kindly curious. When a healthcare provider tells you that, for instance, the periods went away because that's "normal sometimes," it's OK to ask something like, "Is there anything else that could cause this?" That may prompt a healthcare provider to pause and think more broadly about what might be going on.
2. It can also help to send a brief message before the visit with additional background/concerns so that the provider has a heads-up and can plan to check in with you separately, if possible. If you get their reassurance but still feel like something might be going on with your loved one, keep following up so your provider knows that your concerns are ongoing.
3. It's also OK to ask for a second opinion. This may be challenging based on insurance coverage. However, seeking out a medical provider with eating disorder expertise may be needed to get your loved one on the path to recovery.
4. Finally, if you're ever worried about how your child looks (e.g., they're pale, dizzy, fainting, etc.), they should be seen urgently for medical evaluation. Depending on the degree of malnutrition, a missed meal or two, purging, or even exercise may be critical as the body is essentially in survival mode. Make sure to share your concerns about their eating habits so the provider has a full picture about what could be going on.[32]

What if I start to feel concerned or overwhelmed by the initial information?

Those feelings are completely understandable and normal. Please give yourself grace about whatever emotions you're experiencing, and know you are not alone. This is partly why we cannot stress enough the importance of seeking your own support.

Individual therapy can be helpful in processing the feelings and confusions that arise. If you have insurance, check your mental health benefits. If you don't have insurance, there are many generalist practitioners and community agencies that offer sliding scale and pro bono services for individuals in need of financial assistance. (See chapter 6, **What if we can't afford the recommended treatment?** section.)

Most parents are not prepared in advance for an eating disorder (not your fault or theirs) and can find themselves overloaded. Absorb the information as best you can. Notice what makes sense to you and what doesn't. Then, if you can come from a grounded, compassionate stance, feel free to ask your loved one questions, such as

- "I'm curious: What's this like for you?" (or you can pose this as a statement so they feel less pressed to answer, but the door is opened: "I'm interested in what this is like for you.")
- "When do you think this started?"
- "What's the hardest part for you?"

Hopefully, gathering information from them will assuage some of your overwhelm—even if it's just by naming the elephant in the room. Insider's tip: If they're in the beginning stages and not acknowledging having an eating disorder, try something like: "I'm wondering if you think you could have an eating disorder?" Warning: Good chance they'll say no. That's partly because we live in a health-and-thinness-driven culture, and it can be hard to tell exactly when someone's eating disorder develops. Also, people with eating disorders are frequently unable to accurately assess their level of illness and health risks. By asking them questions and reading this book, you're gathering data and being your own citizen scientist.

No matter where you and your loved one are in the process, you're probably trying to start a productive conversation and better understand what's going on. If they react, you may have hit something sensitive. *Just notice.* Try not to panic. Instead, look at what you're learning. You're collecting information for a fuller picture and a better understanding. You're also asking questions because, once you begin to understand the basics of eating disorders, you know there are medical and physical risks that can happen. Those could need attention right away.

Why should I make attending a support group a priority?

While we both try to abstain from using the word *should* (because *should* makes choices into obligations), we intentionally use it here. Of the many things you *could* do next, we believe—in most cases—it will be in your best interest to connect with a support group. We can't tell you how many parents derive a sense of guidance and decreased isolation by attending. A support group will typically introduce you to others who have similar experiences, offer you compassion, keep you privy to current research, share information and tips, and provide a unique sense of community.

Alli witnesses countless touching and beneficial things happen from the support group for caregivers of people with eating disorders that she facilitates:

> People move from feeling "crazy" to feeling validated and understood. I see parents go above and beyond, including helping

out with each other's kids. Group cries happen—laughter, too. Hearts connect.

Support continues outside of the meetings that I facilitate. The members of my group have formed their own text chain. When one wants advice or to practice something challenging, that person texts the others. I often hear about how they show up for each other. Those who live nearby sometimes meet in person.

Group members actively share resources, referrals, and more. Through listening to each other's stories, some have found paths to more effective treatment experiences. A few of those, whose loved ones have healed, continue attending and supporting as a pay it forward to others.

It's one of my favorite things I've done in my career. The love, humility, and dedication that so many parents and caregivers bring is an honor to be in the room (even if it's an online room) with and witness.

In both our practices, we've heard people with eating disorders express relief and hopefulness when their parents are doing their own work. We've seen kids (adult and minor), even those sassy teens, become less defensive and more vulnerable when their parents seek their own support. A caregiver support group can offer benefits for the entire family system.

How do I find a support group?

As of 2025, the following organizations will lead you to active groups and opportunities to connect with other caregivers (in alphabetical order):

Eating Disorder Foundation (EDF)

EDF is a nonprofit organization that is "devoted to helping people with eating disorders, their families and their friends to rebuild shattered lives." EDF currently offers support groups for family and friends.[33]

Families Empowered and Supporting Treatment of Eating Disorders (FEAST)

FEAST is a global nonprofit organization that "walks alongside families as they navigate the challenges of their loved one's eating disorder." FEAST provides parents and caregivers with peer-led support groups and community.[34]

- FEAST's Around the Dinner Table Forum is moderated by experienced caregivers and is specifically for parents and caregivers of loved ones of any age and with any eating disorder.
- Fathers, there is a Men of FEAST group specifically for you. The father of one of Jenny's recovery coaching clients has made lifelong friends from this group. The dads meet in person, golf together, etc. Even now that some of their kids are in a solid place of recovery and they have no need to attend the support group regularly, they stay connected.

International Eating Disorder Family Support (IEDFS)

IEDFS is a "co-ed, peer-to-peer, experienced and EDucated support community" on Facebook that began in 2018. Membership is moderated by parents and other caregivers in the group. Their description specifies, "Since evidence-based protocols and lived [personal] experience are the cornerstone of our support, we welcome discussions of both."[35]

Multi-Service Eating Disorders Association (MEDA)

MEDA is a nonprofit "dedicated to the prevention and treatment of eating disorders." MEDA offers support groups for family and friends.[36]

National Alliance for Eating Disorders (The Alliance)

The Alliance is a nonprofit organization "providing education, referrals, and support for all individuals experiencing eating disorders, as well as their loved ones." The Alliance offers support groups for loved ones of people with eating disorders.[37]

National Association for Anorexia Nervosa and Associated Disorders (ANAD)

ANAD is a nonprofit organization that, according to their website, is the "largest peer support resource for eating disorders in the country." They offer a wide variety of support groups for caregivers.[38]

- There is a sibling support group open to those fifteen years of age and older who have a loved one navigating an eating disorder.
- Alli's support and education group for friends and family of people with eating disorders is listed as an ANAD Affiliate. It's a no-cost group that began in 2011 as a part of the ANAD network.

At the time Alli started her support group, it was one of only a handful of caregiver-focused support groups that existed. (Back when she was going through her eating disorders, there were no readily available parent resources. This is another reason why she feels so passionate about the caregiver community.) Nowadays, many organizations, private practice practitioners, and treatment centers run groups for parents, caregivers, and family members. (Yay!)

To find more options, the internet is your friend. These kinds of support and education groups may be called *friends and family of people with eating disorders support groups*. Other titles may include the terms *for loved ones*, *carers*, *caregivers*, and *parents*. Groups may be

- online or in-person only
- no cost or for a fee
- run by peers
- led by professionals or eating disorders specialists
- requiring regular attendance or allowing drop-in

As you search, check out any groups that seem potentially relevant to your situation. Attending may be the best way to see which might be a fit for you regarding milieu, philosophy, focus, sense of privacy, etc. Once you tap into a support network, you'll probably discover that the people there are tremendously generous with their knowledge and kindness. (We may be biased, though!)

Did I do something to cause the eating disorder?

We understand why this comes up so often. It's natural to want to know.

According to research, cause is quite complicated.[39] For instance, though there are known risk factors (something that increases the likelihood of a disorder or disease developing), no one can predict who will develop an eating disorder. The cause seems to be a complex mix or interplay of biological, environmental, social, and psychological factors. Searching for the cause expends time and energy that could be used more productively. Supporting healing is most important and requires your focus right now.

If you feel guilty and blame yourself for possible mistakes in the past, give yourself some compassion. You were probably doing your best at the time. If there are things you wish you had said or done differently, please forgive yourself and make amends by doing or viewing things differently moving forward.

Could my child die?

Any eating disorder is a disorder that needs to be taken seriously. We encourage you to invest as much time and energy as you possibly can to learn about eating disorders and how you might support your loved one's healing.

And yes, people sometimes die from this illness, but that does not mean your child will. The fact that you are researching, reading, and investing yourself at this point is so helpful and important. Keep learning. Ask questions. Be assertive with treatment providers if needed. And don't give up!

What does it mean to be recovered?

Because we have already used the term recover*ed* (past tense) in the introduction and mentioned "full recovery" earlier in this chapter, we're going to jump into this here and now. You've hit a controversial question: The definition depends on who you ask.

Research has shown that people recovered from eating disorders can be "indistinguishable" from people with no history of eating disorders.[40] To us, that provides a clear example that full recovery is possible. Yet, there is no consensus on the definition of recovered.

In our experience, those who describe themselves as "fully recovered" (and yes, there are many of us out there) usually talk about the freedom that comes from living a life without eating disorder-related thoughts and behaviors—a life they find engaging, meaningful, purposeful, and enjoyable. And this almost necessarily involves at least the criteria described below.

Here's an example of one definition that has received attention in the eating disorder field.[41] Criteria for fully recovered include all the following for at least three months:[42]

1. no longer meeting the *Diagnostic and Statistical Manual of Mental Disorders (DSM)* criteria
2. no binge eating, purging, or fasting
3. a body mass index (BMI) of at least 18.5 (The BMI is a calculation that estimates body fat based on a person's height and weight.)
4. specific score ranges on targeted eating disorder assessments.

It's worth noting that the above is a definition used for research purposes. A study revealed that while some with lived (personal) experience agreed with it, most did not. Issues with the criteria that the recovered participants expressed included duration too short, not comprehensive enough, too absolute, and issues with BMI.[43]

Because every person's eating disorder is experienced uniquely, every person's individual interpretation of recovered/recovery may vary in nuances and priorities. Alli shares some clinical observations:

> For some, they'll add or emphasize what's important to them in their definitions, such as body acceptance, effective coping skills, ability for adulting, better boundaries, more social connection, no longer avoiding being in photographs, or something else. For others, recovered/recovery may mean experiencing fewer to no eating disorder-related thoughts, attitudes, behaviors, and temptations. Recovery goals can change over time.

Without a universally accepted definition of recovered, there's the risk that some may settle for less than the fullest recovery that could be possible for them. For instance, some may believe that the absence of eating disorder behaviors *alone* equates to fully recovered. They could stop there, not pushing for more. *Or*, they could build momentum from accomplishing that and eventually want—and pursue—more freedom from eating disorder-related symptoms. We've witnessed both.

Jenny subscribes to Carolyn Costin's published definition of recovered. As mentioned earlier, Costin not only trained her as a recovery coach but treated her many years ago when she was a client at Costin's treatment facility:

> Being recovered is when the person can accept his or her natural body size and shape and no longer has a self-destructive or unnatural relationship with food or exercise. When you are recovered, food and weight take a proper perspective in your life, and what you weigh is not more important than who you are, in

> fact, actual numbers are of little or no importance at all. When recovered, you will not compromise your health or betray your soul to look a certain way, wear a certain size, or reach a certain number on a scale. When you are recovered, you do not use eating disorder behaviors to deal with, distract from, or cope with other problems.[44]

Jenny shares what this definition looks like and how she got there:

> I no longer have eating disorder thoughts, urges, or behaviors. I have a better relationship to food, exercise, and body than most people who have never even had an eating disorder. For example, I eat when I'm hungry and stop when I'm full. I eat what my body is craving without any judgments or restrictions. Exercise is an outlet and celebration; I move in ways that bring me joy. Physical activity is not a punishment or compensatory behavior. Every so often, I give myself a hug and kiss on the shoulder, telling my body what a good job she is doing. (Insert from Alli: If you think this is b.s., you have not met her!)
>
> Like many, I didn't realize one could be fully recovered (past tense) from an eating disorder until I attended residential treatment at a facility that embraced this concept. Even many of the staff openly identified as being recovered. Before that exposure, I assumed my eating disorder was going to be something I managed my whole life—forever dodging thoughts and urges. It was so helpful for me to know that there were many others who went through eating disorders and came out the other side.

When it comes to your child, we know that you want the best for them—fully recovered. And based on our and many others' experiences, we believe that's likely possible. That said, here's a warning: They may push back, implying that the idea is too lofty or overwhelming right now. In our work, we've seen that some people with eating disorders can find it hopeful and helpful to believe they might someday be completely free of their eating disorder. Others say they find it unhelpful and impossible as an ultimate goal. Instead, they prefer a term or process they feel is more realistic for them, such as healing, improving, in recovery, etc.

Alli shares about her personal healing path:

> After decades of believing my eating disorder was a part of me, I finally wanted its influence to be *less* in my life. Cut to: I ended up recovering, but that was before recover*ed* was considered a possibility. So, when I felt free of the eating disorder, I had nothing to gauge it against. The general belief back then was that eating disorders were life sentences, so the absence of those thoughts, urges, preoccupations, and haunts left me confused.
>
> If the recovered criteria had been presented at any point on my path, would I have eventually gone after it like I went after so many goals in my life? Would I have thought it to be only for others? Would I have skipped over what I could have seen as another set of exhausting rules to pass, fail, or rate myself as "not good enough" at doing? Who knows? What I do know is this: Discovering that the eating disorder *could* be left behind was a huge relief.

Right now, don't get too caught up in the wording your loved one might use about recovery. Do what you need to support any healing momentum. Continue to hold hope for that fully recovered outcome for them, even if they can't fathom that status at this point. Many don't think it's possible for them—even we thought that way about our own healing—and then something shifted.

How long does it take to be recovered?

We understand unknowns can be frustrating, and we wish we could tell you how long it takes. Even research hasn't yet given that answer. A review of over 1,300 studies concluded that "results are difficult to interpret due to inconsistent study definitions of remission, recovery and relapse, lack of longer-term follow-up and the potential for diagnostic crossover,"[45] which is when one eating disorder diagnosis or subtype changes to a different one.

Parents usually want healing and recovery to happen as quickly as possible. Yet the person with the eating disorder often comes at this process from a different space than that. Your loved one may not even want recovery. They may only desire "a little less torment" or to get people "off their back" by agreeing to treatment. (If this sounds like your child, what do they want right now? What are they *willing* to change? That could become a starting point on which to build.)

Enlisting their willingness for the many changes needed to achieve any level of recovery can take time. For instance, nutritional rehabilitation is typically required for your loved one to think more clearly and logically and to nourish their body. Yet, the medicine—regular eating—is the very thing they have a problem doing! So, they are usually conflicted about feeding themselves.

For a while, there could be an ongoing tug-of-war between allowing your child choice and autonomy versus urgent nutritional rehabilitation or medical stabilization. It's tricky! If you feel confused, you're probably right on track.

To get to a place of being fully healed took time for both of us. Our lives grew and evolved as we recovered (e.g., gaining more friends and interests). It felt like a grieving process: You know how after a loss, death, or breakup, some days can feel easier or harder? It was the same with recovery. There was an ebb and flow along the way, but the overall trajectory was one of getting easier as time progressed. (We hear this kind of description over and over from others who have healed.)

Now, please make sure you are sitting down when you read what's next. Some may heal in months, many in years, and others don't ever. It can be a long haul. Research published in 2017—one of the few existing longitudinal studies—indicated that around two-thirds of the females with bulimia nervosa and one-third of females with anorexia nervosa were recovered by a nine-year follow-up, and around two-thirds of both groups were recovered at the twenty-two-year follow-up.[46] That's not to say nine or twenty-two years is the timing. Reminder: The field and science keep making progress. That study began quite a while ago.

Recovery was neither of our goals when we first sought help. Now that we're on the other side, we can't help but want it for the clients we support and their families—no matter how long it takes. Though there are no guarantees, we believe that an important factor will be your meeting your child where they are and trying to move the needle forward.

2

Empathy and Understanding

We acknowledge that the eating disorder's presence can feel both terrifying and infuriating. This chapter aims to facilitate insight and compassion for what your child is going through.

What's it like to have an eating disorder?

This next exercise offers an idea of what it's like to have an eating disorder. Alli created it many years ago. A heads-up: It might feel uncomfortable.

The Experience of an Eating Disorder Exercise

In the last twenty-four hours, have you been to any place where food was not easily available or purchasable?

When presenting workshops on eating disorders, I have asked attendees this question many times. Almost never has anyone reported extended periods of time free of food. Instead, they have shared their surprise at how present and available food is throughout their day, even in places not centered around food: after a religious service, when coffee and donuts are available for people wanting fellowship; at the office supply, home improvement, and hobby stores, snacks surround shoppers in line to check out; at school, a stocked vending machine sits close by; at the airport, mall, etc.

Before proceeding, can you think of any place where food is not nearby?

1. What's something that terrifies you (e.g., snakes, tarantulas, heights, clowns, etc.)?

If you can't find anything that frightens you, then pick something wildly uncomfortable for you. Maybe that's your in-laws, being in tight spaces, public speaking, etc.

2. For the purpose of this exercise, use what you chose wherever it says [my fear] below. Read from start to finish.

At a minimum, I must experience [my fear] four to six times a day (e.g., breakfast, lunch, dinner, and snacks). In addition, no matter where I go throughout the day, [my fear] is usually close by. That could be an advertisement, a smell, or the real thing just a few feet away. Other times it might be invading my personal space, like reaching over [my fear] to pay for something at a checkout register. Or people surprising me with [my fear] as a "treat" or a token demonstrating their affection.

At every party, I'm surrounded by [my fear]. Most get-togethers center on [my fear]. And my friends enjoy and talk about [my fear] while it freaks me out.

Every encounter with [my fear] is just as scary or uncomfortable for me. No amount of repetition makes [my fear] easier or less stressful to experience.

Since I get little to no break from it, I also sometimes obsess about [my fear]. For example, I worry, "When will [my fear] happen next?" I wonder, "How do I avoid [my fear]?" I plot and plan, "How can I hide my reaction to [my fear] so I look normal since most people love [my fear]?"

In the previous statements, [my fear] refers to *food* for someone with an eating disorder.

3. If you were to live this scenario for even seven days in a row, how do you think you'd be feeling right now?

Thank you for doing that exercise. Hopefully, it helped highlight that an eating disorder can be a phobia-like experience splashed with an obsession about the phobia.

What can I do to better understand eating disorders?

Now that you've adjusted to the idea of an eating disorder influencing your child, delving deeper by learning more will likely be in your and your loved one's best interests. Not all major eating disorders nonprofits, websites, or for-profit organizations cater to parents and caregivers, but more do now than they did just a decade ago.

Here, we share some of those major eating disorders nonprofits. Each offers resources that can enhance a caregiver's knowledge of eating disorders, including pamphlets, webinars, podcasts, conferences, and more. All these groups are working around some common goals, albeit with slightly different approaches and offerings, to bring light to the seriousness of eating disorders and often to build community. The nonprofits, with excerpts of their mission statements, and selected examples of their offerings are listed below (in alphabetical order):

Academy for Eating Disorders (AED)

Founded in 1993, "the mission of the AED is to advance eating disorder prevention, education, treatment, and research by expanding the global community of committed professionals."[1] AED offers the following:[2]

- International Conference on Eating Disorders (ICED)

- Resources for Experts by Experience (yes, that means you, parents with personal experience!)
- AED publications, such as
  - *The AED Guide to Selecting Pharmacologic Treatments for Patients with Eating Disorders*
  - *Caregivers: 10 Actions*
  - *Eating Disorders: A Guide to Medical Care*
  - *Eating Disorders in the Emergency Department*
  - *A Guide to Selecting Evidence-Based Psychological Therapies for Eating Disorders*
  - *Guidebook for Nutrition Treatment of Eating Disorders*
  - *Minimum Standards of Care: Cross-Cultural Action Guidelines for Eating Disorders*
  - *Nine More Truths About Eating Disorders: Weight and Weight Stigma*
  - *Nine More Truths About Eating Disorders: Boys and Men*

Families Empowered and Supporting Treatment of Eating Disorders (FEAST)

Formed in 2007, "the mission of F.E.A.S.T. is to walk alongside families as they battle their loved one's eating disorder, providing transformative support, education, empowerment, and community through a multitude of programs and services."[3] FEAST offers the following:[4]

- FEAST of Knowledge Conference
- FEAST Programs, such as
  - FEAST Caregiver Skills Toolkit
  - FEAST 30 Days

Multi-Service Eating Disorders Association (MEDA)

Founded in 1994, "MEDA is dedicated to the prevention and compassionate treatment of eating disorders so that Every Body has access to recovery and support."[5] MEDA offers the following:[6]

- MEDA Recovery Community: free membership for family and friends, which includes access to their online library; select webinars, courses, guided meditations, and recovery tools; and family and friend forums

National Alliance for Eating Disorders (The Alliance)

Founded in 2000, the mission of The Alliance is to provide "education, referrals, and support for all individuals experiencing eating disorders, as well as their loved ones."[7] The Alliance offers the following:[8]

- For Loved Ones section: succinct lists of dos and don'ts and other tips
- Eating Disorders Information Gateway: searchable citation database of books and articles pertaining to eating disorders
- The Alliance Resource Library: brochures, school-focused materials, etc.
- Southern Smash: scale smashing events and SmashTALK panel discussions.

National Center of Excellence for Eating Disorders (NCEED)

Founded in 2018 by the Substance Abuse and Mental Health Services Administration, NCEED's "mission is to advance education and training of healthcare providers and to promote public awareness of eating disorders and eating disorder treatment."[9] NCEED focuses on providing up-to-date, evidence-based information and offers the following:[10]

- Family Members/Friends section: webinars, infographics, etc.

National Eating Disorders Association (NEDA)

Formed in 2001, NEDA "seeks to fundamentally change the way eating disorders are understood and treated so those affected can achieve lasting recovery and well-being."[11] NEDA provides the following:[12]

- Grace Holland Cozine Resource Center: brochures, school-focused materials, etc.
- NEDA Toolkits: for parents, educators, etc.

Project HEAL (PH)

Founded in 2008, the mission of PH is "to break down systemic, healthcare, and financial barriers to eating disorder healing."[13] They offer the following:[14]

- Learn section: information, research, etc.
- PH Recent News and Media Highlights section.

There are many more major eating disorders organizations that focus on information and resources pertinent to their parts of the world. If you are not in the United States, international organizations, such as AED, may be able to direct you. Also, there's good ol' googling.

Please note: Depending on when you read this book, the websites and web pages mentioned might or might not still exist, have merged with another, or been replaced. Things can change quickly in cyberspace. Also, when it comes to information hubs, before wholly trusting, please check for credibility and reputation to the best of your ability.

As you grow your eating disorders education, you'll quickly notice that one source may offer approaches as if they are *the* way. Another provides a different set of instructions—also purporting to be *the* way. People will offer differing views. Some swear by X and others by Y. Even the various official treatment guidelines have limits and are not the be-all and end-all. We firmly believe that the more information you can gather, the better.

Our hope is that your newfound knowledge will give you the background and courage to strategically ask your child more about what they're experiencing (if you have not already). Insider's tip: Your loved one may not understand what's going on for them. So, they may not be able to articulate that for you. However, the following will likely have occurred:

- You learned enough about eating disorders to initiate a thoughtful conversation. (Even if your loved one got upset, yay you!).
- You showed you care.
- You saw them and recognized their struggles while much of society might be complimenting their appearances of discipline, body changes, "healthy" food choices or restraint, etc.
- You opened a door for their self-reflection and your potential understanding.

Eating disorders can conjure up a multitude of negative feelings for you and your loved one alike. Shame, confusion, guilt, self-blame, embarrassment, feeling "stupid," defensiveness, and anger are common experiences. Consequently, people sometimes avoid saying anything at all to their loved one about the eating disorder.

Experience has shown us that's usually a mistake. Why? Saying nothing can look like you don't notice your loved one's experience, unwellness, confusion, struggle, pain, etc. Or you think the eating disorder is OK. (We're pretty sure that's not what you'd want to communicate.)

Why do I feel like I'm walking on eggshells?

Probably because you are. A lot of the time, you can't say anything "right" enough to avoid responses that feel uncomfortable. In our respective roles as therapist and recovery coach, both of us hear this sentiment from parents often. If it matches your experience, you are not the only one.

Here's the good news. When it comes to eating disorders, not knowing and not getting things right are kind of the norm. You're off the hook! Please allow that to comfort you when you hear the crunch of shells under your feet. *(Crunch. Crunch. Crunch.)*

It can be complicated because the person can both desperately want to be seen and helped while being strongly (even forcefully) resistant. Getting a read on them can be difficult; the person may not be able to tell you what they want or need. So for now, you may need to accept that's how it is. But if there's anything disrespectful or abusive going on in your loved ones' responses, that's not OK.

You have a right to live comfortably and be treated with respect in your home. Aside from comments about food, bodies, or exercise, try not to tiptoe because tiptoeing usually gives the eating disorder power. Instead, own your space, meaning be careful of shrinking yourself to accommodate your loved one's moods, whims, demands, etc. And when you say or do the "wrong" thing—notice how we say *when* and not *if*—own it, repair it (if necessary), and move on. And when things go well, make a mental note for future interactions.

Why does it feel as if I no longer know my child?

Because eating disorders can be difficult to comprehend, here is a distant yet likely understood comparison.

- Have you ever been influenced by a friend, significant other, or celebrity idol that your parents didn't totally approve of?
- Did the influence affect how you acted?
- Did it sway your values?

The answer is yes—even if it was only *a little*. (Come on! We're not the only ones who've been there!) Hopefully, you can agree with the general point of the above questions: The influence can make us seem unfamiliar to our loved ones.

Similarly, the eating disorder's influence is likely very different from the core of the person you have known. An eating disorder can make an honest person lie about anything remotely related to eating, exercise, and body image (one's perception of and relationship with their body).

- "I swear I ate," when they didn't
- "No, I didn't eat the last of that," when they did
- "I only worked out a little," when they spent hours and hours
- "I don't like that food," when it used to be their childhood favorite

Alli shares how the eating disorder changed her while she was *in it*:

> Anyone who is close to me would probably attest that I'd rather say something embarrassing or painful than lie. My conscience tears me up about dishonesty because it's against my values. Yet, when I had an eating disorder, I lied about things related to food and exercise. I remember my conscience was not happy. However, protecting the attitudes and behaviors tied to the eating disorder became paramount.

The eating disorder can also bring on dramatic, sudden shifts in the mood or personality of your loved one. A sunshiny kid can turn dark and brooding. A usually kind and gentle child may hiss at you like a feral cat when you ask an innocent question. The unfamiliar *part* of your loved one is likely the eating disorder's influence—at least some of it is, if not all. (And yes, if your child is a teen, it can be challenging to differentiate between what we just described and what's considered "normal" teen behavior.)

Notice we said *part* of your loved one. It's like when someone gets the flu. The flu virus invades and affects the person, and the immune system needs to be strong enough to combat the virus. In the case of an eating disorder, the metaphorical immune system often needs bolstering via support, information, and treatment so it can start to help fight the eating disorder's influence.

Jenny offers her personal experience of what helped her make sense of what was happening within her:

> It links to a concept I was taught both in recovery and as a recovery coach: the eating disorder versus healthy self.[15] The entire time I was sick, there was a split. There were two parts of me. Over time, my eating disorder took over, and I was doing things—like lying, missing class, and flaking on commitments—I would have never

done when I was well. The eating disorder became stronger than the healthy self. However, even in the height of my eating disorder, there was a teeny, tiny part of me that knew some of the things I was doing weren't right, but I wouldn't admit it. For instance, I would have never suggested someone else eat the way I was eating, do the extreme behaviors I was doing, or say the things I was saying to myself to someone else.

I was relieved to learn about the concept of this split. I was so deep in the disorder, I didn't even realize there was a distinction between the two parts of self. It is now a framework I use when coaching my own clients. Some of them use other terms for their healthy self, such as soul self, true nature, wise mind, or even a bad*ss pseudonym. Whatever terminology resonates for the individual.

We recognize that much of what we just described might sound bizarre or even surreal to some. We get that. Not all will relate to the split or parts concepts. Yet, for both of us and numerous folks we've met, the eating disorder seemed like a force that hijacked us—a weird, powerful experience where our normal selves and free will took a backseat to the eating disorder. Bottom line: If your loved one seems like a different person, that could be an important indication that the eating disorder has taken over and is running the show.

Does it make me a bad person if I find myself disliking my child?

Oh goodness, no. You are a person who is going through something very difficult. And that tends to stretch anyone. A lot.

If you spend significant time with your child who has an eating disorder, there is a good chance you will be on the receiving end of their discomfort, distress, or fear at some point(s). As a result, your child may lash out at you, and that feels awful. It is normal to dislike the eating disorder while still loving your child, although it can also be challenging to separate the two.

Taking care of yourself can help you get through this uncomfortableness, which means granting self-compassion. Maybe acknowledge something like the following: "I'm hurt, scared, and angry right now. And it's hard not to feel bad for not liking my child at this moment. I want to like them. I'm sad. I miss them. These are difficult feelings."

OK, OK, we know that sounds super "therapisty." You get the gist. So go ahead and use your own words. But don't be mean to yourself!

Is an eating disorder about wanting to be skinny?

It makes sense why this perception exists, but it is way more complicated than that. Not all eating disorders relate to a desire to be slim. Even the ones that do include a drive for thinness cannot be reduced to "wanting to be skinny."

Some of the main eating disorder diagnoses include a weight focus and self-evaluation linked to body shape or weight, namely anorexia nervosa, bulimia nervosa, and some forms of other specified feeding or eating disorder (OSFED). Others have nothing to do with either per their diagnostic criteria; for instance, binge-eating disorder, avoidant/restrictive food intake disorder (ARFID), and some forms of OSFED. All eating disorders focus on food and eating.

Our society perpetuates weight stigma and thin bias and provides messaging about "healthy eating" reflecting morality (being seen as good/bad due to what we eat). Many people diet for weight or health-related reasons, and that is *often*, but not always, a bridge to an eating disorder's onset.

When Alli discusses cause, she likens the eating disorder to a metaphorical on/off button. It simply exists in some people, likely due to genetics. Usually, no one is aware it's there. Then, something or a bunch of things happen—psychological and physiological vulnerabilities and risk factors[16]—that push the button on.

There are many aspects not initially related to wanting to be skinny that may activate the development of an eating disorder. For instance, someone experiences being bullied, cyberbullied, or teased and reacts by emotional eating, bingeing, or restricting.[17] Someone else attempts to address health issues by eliminating certain foods or food groups (e.g., carbs, sugar, wheat, fat, or animal products). Still another, upon a medical professional's advice, sets forth to change their diet or lose weight for better longevity. And yet another faces an illness, like cancer, which temporarily disrupts their eating patterns, appetite, and emotional equilibrium.[18] Yes, those are all real examples.

Once the metaphorical eating disorder button is on, various psychological reasons and secondary gains (the benefits of remaining sick) contribute to the persistence of the eating disorder. Some experience the eating disorder as a way to

- cope
- fit in socially (by changing their body to one that feels safer, more desirable, or more accepted)
- distract from uncomfortable or scary life stressors
- create structure (with reliability, organization, and predictability)
- provide a sense of autonomy or identity

- become more confident (if or when they can reach some food or body-related goal)
- suppress sexuality and unwanted sexual objectification
- receive positive praise and attention (The person tends to be showered with "You lost weight. You look great," "You're so disciplined," and "I wish I could eat like you." The irony is they might binge in private, often *cannot* eat anything they deem as "unhealthy" or "less healthy" than something else, etc.)
- feel special
- substitute for emotions (i.e., focusing on the feeling of an empty stomach may be more tolerable than feeling emotions)
- attempt to halt maturation that they didn't believe they were ready for, particularly in early adolescence
- and more.

Let us stress: Your loved one is generally not consciously manipulating you or mindfully choosing the above. They're usually doing their best to simply live their lives.

Jenny provides some real-life examples, ranging from her recovery coaching clients to herself:

> I've had clients who, after their disorder began, discovered a myriad of secondary gains—even if the disorder started as an attempt to achieve thinness. As an example, I worked with a teen whose father was heavily involved in her sibling's athletic activities. However, when she got sick, the father often skipped practices or games to make sure she was eating her food. Ultimately, she discovered and was able to share that she was scared of getting better. Why? Because it would mean less time and attention from her father. None of this was consciously or actively manipulative on her part.

I worked with an adult client who was financially dependent on her parents. Living independently felt overwhelming, and she didn't trust herself to do it well. Her eating disorder postponed her mastering bills, work, school, and expectations in general. Again, this was not an intentional avoidance.

Still, I had another adolescent client whose eating disorder was a big F'-you to her parents' own food rules. She was forced to eat one way at her mother's house and a completely different way at her father's house. She didn't know how to fight back to defend her food autonomy (being able to make one's own choices about what and when to eat). Until she could learn how to set boundaries, not eating was the best she could do to take care of herself.

In my own story, the dynamics in my family were tumultuous. The eating disorder was a coping method—albeit a dangerous one—that served me while I was in a toxic environment.

When I look back, my eating disorder gave me something to focus on that let me distract from the chaos I was experiencing. Purging and exercise were like pressure release valves. It's hard to explain, but as it nearly killed me, it oddly helped me get through until I could be introduced to people (providers) who could show me a healthier way of coping.

We hope that these examples help you to take in something counterintuitive: how the eating disorder can feel subjectively helpful or beneficial to the person while objectively harming them.

Not all treatment providers stress exploring these kinds of secondary gains and maintaining factors. Still, from our experience, we believe that people with eating disorders can benefit from unpacking these wants and needs as a part of therapy, seeing if they can get them met in different, sustainable, non-eating disordered ways.

Are eating disorders fueled by vanity?

Though this question is similar to the above, we included it because it's a common myth out there. We understand that at times, the eating disorder makes a person seem vain or hyper-focused on their looks. You may notice something referred to as body checking, which may manifest as staring in the mirror, taking selfies, trying on specific-sized clothes, gazing at their window reflections, or scrutinizing their body in other creative ways. But here, body checking is not a sign of self-admiration.

Many with eating disorders (not all) have body distortions. They can genuinely see something like you might see in a carnival funhouse mirror. Though their glancing might look self-absorbed, they could actually be seeking reassurance while scared that something has changed massively since the last time they checked. But no, neither of us has ever seen "vanity" as the exclusive reason for an eating disorder. It typically goes much, much deeper.

Are eating disorders about needing control?

We worry about the ongoing perpetuation of the "control" interpretation. It's way too simple an explanation for what's behind eating disorders (or any psychological disorder, for that matter). We hear it often—even from those who have recovered: "My eating disorder was about control." And while that may be true to some extent, it is often a narrative that they latched onto after hearing it from a health professional or the media. One of the major problems of the control narrative is how it is frequently interpreted by the person with the eating disorder.

We—and probably anyone who knows someone with an eating disorder—have noticed that people with eating disorders often have poor self-esteem, which research supports.[19] That control narrative can make it worse. "Great, now I'm a controlling person, too." This is a paraphrase, but a repeated sentiment heard in Alli's practice. She explains, "In my clinical experience, they've typically been seeking safety and predictability when their lives or their inner worlds felt otherwise unpredictable, scary, or chaotic."

Believing that eating disorders are only, or even mainly, about control could stop someone from addressing what's actually happening and needing attention. It may be worth an exploration of "it's about control" before buying into it as *the* explanation.

Why can't they just stop their destructive behavior(s)?

Stop what? Bingeing? Restricting? Excessive movement? Their beliefs about food, eating, and exercise? The short answer is that they have a psychological *illness* that makes discontinuing those difficult. Beyond that, it's complicated. Currently, there is no single answer as to why someone cannot simply stop. However, what is clear from clinicians, researchers, and people with eating disorders is that the thoughts and behaviors can be persistent and highly resistant to change.[20] There are a number of factors that have been identified as contributing to the difficulty of discontinuing these behaviors. There are various psychological reasons and secondary gains that can make behavior change difficult, which were discussed earlier in this chapter. (See the **Is an eating disorder about wanting to be skinny?** section.) Further, science continues to uncover biological and brain-related reasons why eating disorders may be so hard to shut down. A variety of potential examples follow, ranging from the effects of insufficient nutrition to more purely neurobiological factors.

Insufficient nutrition can be a part of any eating disorder that restricts intake; for example, anorexia nervosa; atypical anorexia nervosa, which is anorexia nervosa without an underweight body mass index (BMI); avoidant/restrictive food intake disorder (ARFID); and at times, bulimia nervosa. Even among those without eating disorders, insufficient nutrition can *cause* eating disorder-like symptoms.[21] Examples follow:

- If we—any of us—undereat, our bodies may force us to overeat or binge. It's a biologically driven binge. When connected with an eating disorder, the person typically undereats again to compensate for the binge, and the cycle repeats.
- Insufficient nutrition can result in a preoccupation or obsession with food (e.g., cooking, thinking about food, dreaming about it, reading recipes, discussing it, watching cooking shows, watching others eat, etc.). When tied to an eating disorder, a lack of or unbalanced nourishment can intensify the existing preoccupations and obsessions.

The effects of undernutrition can keep people with eating disorders *stuck* and repeating their behaviors.

Some bodies have an opposite response to hunger. Instead of becoming hangry (a blend of hunger and anger), they feel calmer or better.[22] For these folks, consuming an appropriate, "normal" amount of food can lead to increased anxiety and discomfort within themselves. Let's say you have an anxious temperament: Wouldn't you want to feel calmer inside? The anxiety-reducing effect of undereating may lead some people to self-medicate, making them vulnerable to patterns of undereating found in restrictive eating disorders.

Interoception awareness is "the act of consciously sensing, interpreting, and integrating information about the state of inner body systems," such as hunger, fullness, thirst, heartbeat, and internal pain.[23] Research shows that problems with interoception (the body's internal sensory system) are associated with disordered eating, seem to be experienced across eating disorder types, and may contribute to the maintenance of eating disorders.[24] Consider this: How can one take care of even basic needs (e.g., eating) when the cues in their brains and bodies can't be properly read or trusted? Thankfully, research backs the idea that interoception can improve.[25]

Neuroscience explains the complex process of habit formation. In short—while simplified here—the brain determines when something is practiced enough to become automatic. The individual doesn't consciously make that choice. Eating disorder beliefs and behaviors can become habits, occurring involuntarily, as if on autopilot.

Consider when you've first adopted a new belief or behavior. A habit begins to form. Initially, this takes energy and effort. At some point, when the thought or behavior becomes repeated and well-practiced enough, voila! You've formed a new habit! We *all* probably know firsthand how challenging it can be to break habits.

There seems to be a relationship between reward pathways (e.g., dopamine) and binge eating—a complicated relationship, but a relationship nonetheless.[26] For some people, eating a lot at once can provide a pop of euphoria—think retail therapy or winning money in Vegas. Get the picture? That probably contributes to the difficulty in stopping the binge eating involved in certain eating disorders. The range of other factors is broad, and changes in the brain's structure can happen during eating disorders.[27] The most crucial point here is that sometimes the brain overrides the individual's choice and logic, keeping your loved one semi-trapped in a cycle of eating disordered behaviors and beliefs.

Bottom line: Why your loved one can't "just stop" their eating disorder-related beliefs and behaviors is partially because of maintaining factors (influences that support the continuation or worsening of mental health issues) that keep it going. Those cycles tend to need interrupting and at least some correcting before more symptoms and underlying issues can be addressed meaningfully.

Having so many self-perpetuating maintenance factors can feel almost insurmountable to a person with an eating disorder. Yet many break the cycles and heal. Jenny offers what got her unstuck:

> When I was in my eating disorder, I was starving, both literally and metaphorically. It wasn't until I was in treatment for some time that I realized my emotional hunger scared me even more than my physical hunger. I thought my needs were too great to be met and would scare others away. Funny, because I also had internalized the belief: *You're not enough.* Try finding a solution for being too much and not enough at the same time . . . enter anorexia nervosa.
>
> The loving symptom interruptions I received during treatment were profound. The staff at the residential ate with me at meals and stayed with me afterward to make sure I didn't use compensatory behaviors. They comforted me with compassion as I sobbed my way through not being able to use my eating disorder to cope. They helped me grocery shop, cook, and portion my food in a manner that supported recovery. Exposure to exercise was supervised, and feelings that came up around stopping after an appropriate amount of time were explored.
>
> It's hard to explain, but I felt cared for in a way I never had before. It was a turning point. It wasn't a quick fix or cure, but it was the start of a path towards healing.

What helps people to interrupt or stop using eating disorder behaviors will have some commonalities, like nourishment can be key. Yet you can expect some differences, too. For instance, Alli didn't have access to the level of support Jenny received, and she, too, was able to get unstuck. What's important here is the *possibility* and *hope* that your loved one will eventually be able to stop.

What if my loved one feels they are in the wrong body?

Could it mean they wish they had a different figure or physique—as in they're comparing? Sure. Could it mean their body does not feel safe because there was something bad or traumatic that happened to it? Yes. But it can also mean something different: gender dysphoria (the distress of being in a body that does not align with one's gender identity or expression).

We reached out to a colleague with both professional and lived (personal) experience to discuss what it means and how gender dysphoria might play into eating disorders. Jess Hudgens, MA, LPC, LCMHC, ASDCS, NCC, is a queer, neurodivergent therapist who has worked in the eating disorder field for over a decade. Her/their biggest passion is social justice. Jess is a university counselor and often works with individuals who are struggling with both eating disorders and gender dysphoria. She shares this:

> A lot of times, the eating disorder provides a way to disconnect from the body, making it easier to get through the day when every moment feels excruciating because your body doesn't feel like *you*. This emerged as a primary theme in recent research about the connections between eating concerns in trans and nonbinary

individuals[28]—eating forces us to *connect* to our bodies in ways that are inherently uncomfortable if we are experiencing gender dysphoria. This isn't to say that every trans, nonbinary, or gender non-conforming person with an eating disorder has chosen disordered eating patterns to deal with this distress.

It's also possible that the disordered behaviors have their origins elsewhere but provide relief from the gender dysphoria due to the minimization or elimination of secondary sex characteristics (those physical characteristics that arise during puberty such as breasts, menstruation, genital and facial hair, etc.). My dysphoria tends to be most highly triggered by menstruation, so restricting provided a way to eliminate this (along with my breasts, hips, and other things that marked me as "female"). For those assigned male at birth, an eating disorder and hormonal changes might mean minimizing facial hair or the deepness of their voice, or lessening sexual arousal that increases bottom dysphoria.

The connections between your loved one's disordered eating and their experience of their body may work in either direction—and your loved one may not even realize the connections until sometime in their recovery process (this was certainly true for me!). So even if your person hasn't expressed discontent with their gender before, if you hear them state that they feel like they are in the "wrong" body, be curious about what they mean and how they feel about the body they're in. Ask if there are aspects of their bodies that feel wrong, what about them feels wrong, and seek out support for your loved one (and yourself) if warranted.[29]

If a version of Jess's story might be occurring for your loved one, we encourage you to seek a qualified professional who understands both eating disorders and gender dysphoria. Look for the current terms, *gender-affirming* and *body-affirming care.*

I'm told what I shouldn't say, but what should I say?

You *"should"* stop saying *"but"* and *"should."* (Ha ha! We made a funny!)

In all seriousness, how did that feel to be told what to do in the above sentence? Pressuring, right? Like now you *fail* if you say "but" or "should."

"Should" statements can take away or diminish anyone's sense of autonomy. "You should try this." "You should solve your problem by . . ." These kinds of declarations may cause your loved one to feel as if they fail or let you down if they don't do or agree with your "should."

Throughout the years, we've noticed that many people with eating disorders have called themselves "people-pleasers." Research supports that this could be a trend in females, in particular, with eating disorders.[30] That means not being able to follow through on your "should" could cause significant distress for your loved one. So if you can be mindful and strategic about when you use "should," it will probably benefit both you and your loved one.

And about "but," consider this sentence fragment: "You are a wonderful person, but . . ." The minute the *but* comes in, the whole first half is gone. Right? "I like you, but . . ." Though it's grammatically incorrect, sometimes, "and" is way better to use if you want to be heard. "You are a wonderful person, and . . ." "I like you, and . . ."

In general, open-ended and process-oriented questions (questions you cannot answer yes/no) tend to help your loved one grow and realize more about what's going on inside for them. These questions are also likely to give you more information and perspective about what they are experiencing. Even if they snap at you, you still asked. That matters.

Here is a list of helpful phrases that we've seen create effective communication when talking to someone with an eating disorder.

- "I'm curious, what's that like?"
- "What do you think? And it's OK if you don't know."
- "I have ideas, and I'd love to hear your thoughts first."
- "How do you feel about that?"
- Using "I hear" or "I see" with "that this is hard for you" can feel more empathetic than "I know this is hard for you." It reflects that you are paying attention to their experience.

Communicating with your child may feel difficult during an eating disorder. To make that easier, you might add tools to your communication toolbox for sparking motivation, bolstering boundary setting, etc. Here are some online resources other parents have found helpful:

- Codependents Anonymous (CoDA) is a fellowship whose "only requirement for membership is a desire for healthy & loving relationships."[31]
- Emotion-Focused Family Therapy (EFFT) is "a community-based model rooted in principles of anti-oppression and a deep and unwavering belief in the healing power of families and systems, the essence of EFFT is to afford caregivers and significant others a key role in supporting their loved one's mental health and well-being."[32] Currently, there are various free instructional videos for EFFT online at Mental Health Foundations.[33] The approach was created for eating disorders work.
- Nonviolent Communication (NVC) is a "way of being in the world" where "the purpose is to serve life and to create

connection in such a way that everyone's needs can be met through natural care."[34]

Finally, if you can, find a support group for friends and family of people with eating disorders. That can also help aid you with communication skills. (See chapter 1, **How do I find a support group?** section.)

You have a right to speak your truth, and how you say it will matter. (Notice how we used "and" and didn't use "but" there?)

Will we ever get the kid we knew and loved back?

We understand why you might wonder that. When it comes to eating disorders, terrific, core parts of your loved one *seem* to go away, but rest assured, they don't. Here's what we mean. Please read the following as a dialogue:

Alli: Hey, Jenny. What would people say is awesome about you?

Jenny: I'm precise, thorough, high energy, and determined.

Alli: How have those traits served you and hurt you?

Jenny: At best, those traits kept me excelling academically, involved in various extracurricular activities, and out of trouble. At worst, those same traits caused me to be perfectionistic, obsessive, anxious, and stubborn.

Alli: Ahhh. Got it.

Jenny: My precision, thoroughness, high energy, and determined nature—when not channeled in the right direction—brought about panic attacks, made it difficult to connect with peers, and kept me entrapped in the chains of an eating disorder.

Jenny continues to paint a picture for you:

> As you can probably imagine, with the traits I mentioned, I was a natural-born rule follower. Accordingly, I believed I had no other choice than to obey the arbitrary rules of my eating disorder; any deviation resulted in self-punishment. But these were some sick, twisted rules I was now beholden to. I was a girl obsessed. Obsessed not with a boy, but with calories, miles run, pounds/inches lost, the size of my pants, and having perfect skin, hair, make-up, and nails to mask how sick it was making me. I was a shell of my former self, on autopilot with no means of stopping without serious intervention.
>
> However, through recovery, not only did my loved ones "get me back," but I got myself back—and a more resilient version, at that.

Hopefully, that example helps you to know that your loved one is still in there. Here's a question Alli has used in her clinical work to help clients understand this concept.

> I ask them to name a trait that makes them good at their eating disorder. They often reply with something in the vein of, "I'm manipulative," or "You have to be good at manipulating people." To that, I say, "OK, and what is manipulative really? Is it the ability to get others to agree with you? To get them on your side and even do what you want?" There's usually a nod of agreement that communicates a skeptical, "Where are we going with this?"
>
> "So you're persuasive. And isn't that a great trait in a leader? Maybe on a job resume? In politics?" Another nod usually comes.
>
> Then, I explain that the eating disorder is using up that persuasiveness—along with many other talents and gifts—for its benefit. Once the eating disorder is less powerful, those attributes

will be freed up and able to be applied elsewhere in life, like social, professional, and creative realms. At this point, their facial expression usually softens.

Your loved one's characteristics are being used as liabilities instead of assets.[35] For all the *Star Wars* fans out there: Think Anakin Skywalker to Darth Vader.[36]

You may prefer a different contextualization: superpowers used for good versus evil, beneficial versus detrimental, harmful versus helpful, recovery-minded versus eating disordered, etc. Whichever resonates most, go for it! We believe this framing provides an understanding of why you might feel like you've lost your kid, and that it is, indeed, very possible that you will get them back. Insider's tip: We have to be honest, just as anyone who goes through something difficult and heals from it, parts of them will probably be changed and more evolved. You've loved them at every stage of growth so far, and this will be another.

3

Cultural Myths and Messages

Our relationships to food, body, and movement fall somewhere on a spectrum that ranges from nothing problematic to a full-blown eating disorder. This chapter explores societal attitudes and behaviors that can affect your loved one's healing.

Isn't being thin always a good thing?

No, not always. It makes sense you might think that, given that we live in a society of diet culture with consistent covert and overt messaging. Diet culture favors thinness as *the* ideal and automatically healthy.

You'll probably hear the phrase "diet culture" a lot while your loved one is in the process of healing. That is because most eating disorders take some aspects of diet culture to extremes. Those may include, but are not limited to, the following:

- equating healthy/unhealthy statuses with body size
- labeling foods as "good" or "bad"

- counting calories
- tracking macros (macronutrients, the essential nutrients that provide energy to the body)
- eliminating or restricting entire food groups (e.g., fats, carbs, dairy)
- exercising to compensate for eating
- being on the anti-cellulite bandwagon of freezing, creams, etc.
- having biases about people due to their weight, shape, eating styles, body composition, etc.

While we're all steeped in the cultural messages about thinness, not everyone develops an eating disorder. Some people can live their lives according to diet culture without significant consequences. Others may exhibit disordered eating patterns. And then there are those who develop clinical eating disorders. For the last group, full recovery usually requires a shift in perspective, values, and priorities around food and eating, which means no longer subscribing to diet culture and its mandates—or, at the very least, subscribing a heck of a lot less. Parents, that applies to you, too.

If we almost lost you in the prior sentence, we get it. We understand that ditching diet culture mentality can be difficult for some. While you don't *have* to dump it altogether for your child to recover, it could be one of the most supportive and impactful things you do.

Aren't eating disorders a girl's thing?

People of all genders can struggle with eating disorders.

Historically, most cases of eating disorders were described in females. Thus, decades of studies have focused primarily on that group, and as a result, there was likely a reinforcing cycle where clinicians and researchers weren't looking for eating disorders in other genders. Even amenorrhea (a loss of one's period) was a criterion for anorexia nervosa that wasn't removed until 2013 in the *Diagnostic and Statistical Manual of Mental Disorders, Fifth Edition (DSM-5).* So the misconception that eating disorders are a girls' thing makes sense, but it isn't reality.

Men and boys have been in the shadows when it comes to eating disorders treatment and research. For instance, the residential level of care has only been available to them since 1997. Yet research shows that males may account for approximately twenty percent of those with anorexia nervosa, thirty percent of those with bulimia nervosa, forty-three percent of those with binge-eating disorder, and fifty-five to seventy-seven percent of those with other specified feeding or eating disorder (OSFED).[1] Data on avoidant/restrictive food intake disorder (ARFID) is emerging; in one study, males comprised thirty-six percent of adolescents and young adults with that diagnosis.[2]

Males may present with symptoms that match existing criteria (e.g., bingeing, purging, striving for thinness, overvaluation of weight and shape, etc.). And they may not. For instance, what about those who don't restrict for weight loss but to build lean mass?

Consider the "idealized" male physique. In pursuit of it, there can be an intense focus on musculature (e.g., ripped abs, bulking up, etc.) and body composition. Many of the existing eating disorders assessments can't detect those kinds of attitudes and related behaviors.[3] Pursuit of a muscly, cut body is also becoming increasingly common among women and girls who subscribe to the fitness influencer aesthetic.[4]

People who identify as gender nonbinary or gender expansive (genders other than male and female) experience eating disorders, too. In fact, data thus far reveals that transgender people, for example, seem even more vulnerable to eating disorder symptomatology than cisgender people (people who identify with the gender assigned to them at birth).[5]

As challenging as it can be for anyone who is struggling to ask for help, being underrepresented in the literature and underrecognized in the population has created barriers to accessing treatment.[6] Thankfully, the field is evolving in this area.

Isn't my child too old to develop an eating disorder?

These disorders can develop or reemerge at *any* age—from childhood to teens, to early adulthood, to midlife, to later life, to the elderly. The National Institute of Mental Health lists the midpoint age of onset for anorexia nervosa and bulimia nervosa as eighteen and for binge-eating disorder as twenty-one.[7]

There has been an uptick in older adults seeking treatment for late-onset and preexisting eating disorders.[8] Periods of significant transition or change (divorce, children leaving home, major relocations, pregnancy, parenthood) may increase vulnerability to the development or reemergence of eating disorder symptoms.[9] We're also talking about the menopause transition time. One explanation might be that some have a vulnerability to eating disorders during significant hormonal changes.[10]

Just because transitions in life seem to be a vulnerability for eating disorders, please don't fret! We know many recovered folks who have made it through major transitions—even menopause—without relapsing. Alli is included. Her menopausal transition lasted well over a decade. She shares,

It was wild! I'm talking about the hot flashes, mood swings, irritability, night sweats, digestion changes, loss of strength, and more. My mind got cloudy; I began experiencing confusion and distractibility. My body's shape and texture seemed to change overnight. I had no control over any of it.

I was fortunate to know what aging does to a woman's body. Growing up, a medical provider had posters in her office that taught about the changes occurring in each decade. So I didn't seriously contemplate fighting with Mother Nature about any of it.

I think that the hardest part of the peri and menopause periods was feeling alone. I wish women talked to each other more about this stuff. It felt pretty jarring at times. I can see how experiencing so much change (hormonally, physically, appearance-wise, and psychologically) could make someone vulnerable to a lot of things, not to mention an eating disorder.

We wish we could assure you that age alone protects a person from developing an eating disorder, exacerbating a preexisting one, or triggering a relapse. But not necessarily. To answer your question clearly, no, your child is not too old to develop an eating disorder.

Why isn't the body mass index an accurate gauge of health?

The body mass index (BMI) calculation was developed in the 1830s by a Belgian statistician interested in the "normal" man. In the 1970s, a physiologist and researcher built on the original principles and emphasized its usefulness in data analysis in population studies.[11] Notice a trend? The BMI wasn't designed to be a measure of individual health, and it wasn't designed by medical professionals. On the most basic level, the BMI is a mathematical equation that doesn't account for bone density, muscle versus fat weight, or other markers of health. Think about the fact that Olympic athletes have landed in the overweight and obese categories of the BMI.[12] It is not as reliable as Western medicine often promotes. (Don't believe it? "Top 10 Reasons Why the BMI is Bogus," released by National Public Radio, is a quick read packed with information.)[13]

Some people are only able to reach the BMI weight category of healthy/normal when they're sick with an eating disorder, using drugs, battling cancer, or dealing with something else awful and unhealthy. Ironic, since that category is typically conflated with being healthy.

When it comes to eating disorders, the BMI can be particularly misleading as a gauge of wellness. Someone with atypical anorexia nervosa or another form of other specified feeding or eating disorder (OSFED), binge-eating disorder, bulimia nervosa, or unspecified feeding or eating disorder (UFED) might land in that idealized healthy/normal BMI category, making their eating disorder invisible to anyone simply recording the BMI. And someone with an eating disorder whose weight puts them in the BMI category of overweight or obese will often be advised to lose weight to improve their health status, per the BMI, further exacerbating their eating disorder.

Doesn't everyone stress over what they eat or how they look?

Unfortunately, cultural messaging places a great amount of value on what we each eat and how we each look. That has led to a normalization of being critical of our bodies, eating habits, and looks. However, no, not everyone stresses about food or their appearance. Though we must confess that when we meet someone who has not *ever* been touched by societal pressures, we're slightly awed.

My child isn't underweight, so how can they be sick?

People of any weight can have an eating disorder.

During the years that Alli directed #ShakeIt for Self-Acceptance!,[14] a series of public mental health events centered on a flash mob dance (that's where a group of people unexpectedly break into a choreographed dance in public), people asked her how she was going to handle the "super skinny," "anorexic-looking" participants. Would they be allowed to dance? She used those moments to educate with her reply: The average-size or curvy person standing next to them may be the one who's sicker and medically compromised.

We don't have X-ray vision of anybody's status, from healthy to unhealthy, nourished to malnourished, and mental wellness to unwellness. Anorexia nervosa has received a ton of media attention partly because of the spectacle of über-thinness. Yet people who look "healthy" or who might be called "overweight" can be as sick or sicker (e.g., from restricting their food) than the person who you think looks "scary-thin."

Unfortunately, a person's weight and body mass index (BMI) are often used as primary indicators of wellness and illness when it comes to eating disorders. Most health insurance providers emphasize them in their treatment guidelines. Same with many major practice guidelines that doctors, therapists, and dietitians typically consult.

People may be denied care based on their weight or BMI, or their insurance stops paying once they reach a weight or BMI that is no longer deemed dangerous by these outside forces—even though their mind is often still just as sick, if not sicker. In this numbers-focused way, the system perpetuates the recovery-relapse cycle so prevalent with eating disorders.

Please don't get caught up in looks or weight indicating sickness or wellness at a glance. Not only does that reinforce harmful stereotypes, but it can also create a sense of false reassurance and/or unnecessary concern when judging health based on weight.

Will my child have to gain weight to recover?

We've heard this question a lot of times, and people ask it for different reasons. From what we've witnessed, our best answer is maybe, and maybe not. It will depend on their body's needs to function maximally. That applies to a person of any size.

If someone is using eating disorder behaviors to maintain a certain body shape or size, you can most likely anticipate that those behaviors are going to have to change in order to recover. If your child is under their optimal weight, then the answer is probably yes, they will have to gain weight to recover. There may be additional factors at play, such as if they're still growing, heredity, how suppressed their weight is, etc.

We can understand wanting to protect your loved one from the discomfort they might feel from a changed body shape and size. We can also understand that you may have your own ideas about ideal body shapes and sizes. Let's cut to the chase: If you are worried about their body or attractiveness even remotely, then your child's healing may benefit from you doing some work on internal bias about weight. In your defense, you have been indoctrinated into a society that is laden with fatphobia—it's nearly impossible not to have some biases simply due to the world we all live in and cultural messages.

Do I need to stop telling my child they're beautiful or handsome?

If you do it frequently, here's why you may want to stop, at least for now. While for some people with eating disorders, it can be flattering to receive appearance-based compliments, for others, it can build pressure and stress them out.

Alli shares her thoughts as a therapist:

> Throughout the years, I've often heard parents say, in front of their kids, things like, "She's a looker!" "He's so handsome," "They're gorgeous," etc. Though well-intended, I suspect that these looks-based comments come with some danger. Here's what I mean, so you can manage it as you best see fit.
>
> Thus far, I've not met anyone with an eating disorder who didn't seem activated by appearance comments. Even *compliments* can be misinterpreted as *my looks ARE my value*. I'm not sure whether it's the effects of the wonky nutrition, sensitive temperaments to begin with, or something else.
>
> At least during the early recovery stages, can you consider not doing it or try to compliment in ways that deemphasize physical attractiveness but still express your enthusiasm and appreciation? For instance, if you think they look great, instead of "You look beautiful/handsome/pretty," get specific about why, in that moment, you felt an impulse to compliment them. You might say, "I love your style," "Sharp outfit!" "Your eyes are so bright," "You look so fancy!" etc. See how those are different but continue to convey your admiration and enthusiasm?

Jenny shares her experience and perspective:

> It may be worth asking what it's like for them to receive comments about their appearance. I have had recovery coaching clients share that they do appreciate external validation (myself included). And when they don't receive any feedback, they question if they're an "ogre."

Since you might be feeling like you're in a pickle, here's help: If you find yourself praising your child's physical appearance, make sure you are also validating internal traits as well.

What characteristics do you value about your loved one? Absolutely, comment on those! "You are so smart, caring, talented, responsible, tenacious, articulate, loyal, honest, etc." "That was such a kind thing to do." "I appreciate your thoughtfulness." You get the picture. Those kinds of comments help them know more about their worth outside of looks. Even if they try to dismiss this kind of feedback, it's important for them to hear that you value not just *what* they look like, but *who* they are.

On that note, we've noticed that praise focused on performance (e.g., "Great job!" "You'll ace it." "You always do great.") can be similarly misheard. People with eating disorders tend to have black/white and good/bad thinking, with little to nothing in between.[15] There's a chance that your loved one might misconstrue what you're communicating regarding performance-type comments. Alli illustrates this point with a brief personal story:

> When my own parents said, "Just do your best, Alli," I recall feeling pressured. I reasoned, "Well, that's one hundred percent. Straight A's only. That's what 'best' means."
>
> Ummm, that was not what they meant. They meant it to take stress *off* me! Yet I moved forward, pressuring myself with what translated to "Work to get one hundred percent on everything."

I berated myself when I fell short. For example, I remember being filled with disgust and shame, saying that a B was a horrible letter for me to receive as a grade. This was not a realistic way to live; I was too embarrassed to tell anyone, so I just worked harder.

As years passed, I was either doing "my best" or I believed I failed. There was little to nothing in between the two. (Thank goodness for growth and not living that way anymore.)

Yes, we just threw eggshells on your floor. *(Crunch. Crunch. Crunch.)*

A way to step off those eggshells is to ask about your child's experience and remind them that their worth isn't equal to their achievements. Instead of (or in addition to) "Great job!" how about something like the following?

- "How do you feel?" This is a potential gauge question. (Let's say their response is "Happy," "Bummed it's over," "Exhausted," or "Disappointed I didn't do better." See how their answer will probably provide you with valuable information?)
- "I'm curious, what was your process like on the way to that award?" and then "What was easy for you? More challenging?" (This inquiry lets you into more of their process and allows them to know you care about that process, too—not just the product.)
- "What do you think getting all A's gives to you? What about what it takes from you?" (Again, you're communicating interest about more than the result.)
- "No matter what you achieve or don't achieve, I love you to the moon and back." (Here it's just a reminder that their worth is steady, despite excelling, failing, or anything in between.)
- "It's great you got such high grades. And I care most that you're learning and enjoying yourself." (We like this because it

reminds them of what's most important *to* you and *for* them—their process of learning and their enjoyment in it.)

If you disagree with this section or think we are nitpicking, we get it. You may feel it's too much. Maybe you worry, "What if my kid never hears they're attractive?" "What if they never hear they did a great job?" OK, those could be valid concerns, too. Even so, we're confident that this type of protective thoughtfulness will help many people with eating disorders out there.

How do I know if my food, exercise, or body image is affecting them?

You could start by simply asking them. Sometimes that works. *If* they answer, you could be surprised at what's considered problematic or triggering (activating). It might not be anything obvious to you. Or, you may not get their *real* truth. Some (many, in our experience) won't be able to answer or will hold back. We encourage you to assume that your own relationship to food, exercise, and body image will affect them to some degree, be it positively or negatively.

With that said, let's start by exploring your relationship with food by asking yourself:

- How do I talk about food (tastes, what I will eat next, etc.)?
- Am I flexible, or do I have rigid rules about my food?
- Do my words give food neutrality (all foods fit, there are no bad foods) or moral values (healthy/unhealthy, good/bad)?

Next, consider your relationship with movement and exercise:

- Am I flexible, or do I have rigid rules about exercise?
- Do I feel preoccupied or upset when I miss a workout?

- Is my exercise motivated by earning or working off food?
- Do I say "I'm bad" if I don't exercise or "I'm good" if I do?

Finally, take a moment to reflect on body image:

- How do I talk about my body or other people's bodies?
- Do I feel preoccupied or distressed by my shape, size, or weight?
- Do I talk about bodies in a way that objectifies or communicates desirability and undesirability (e.g., "good body," "would be attractive if . . ." "gorgeous legs," "look how tiny they are!" etc.)?

Your attitudes, comments, and behaviors have the potential to activate, amplify, and align with eating disorder thinking—or challenge it.

For people with eating disorders, focusing on others' bodies, food, and exercise (this includes their family members) is quite common.[16] Many of our past therapy and recovery coaching clients have confided about how triggering their parents' eating and exercise patterns feel, including what they talk about.

Comments about how full you are, how much you ate, or how little you exercise and thus feel guilty can derail their progress. We suggest staying away from discussions about food, body, and/or exercise—especially at mealtimes and as best as you can. Ultimately, in eating disorder recovery, talking about your body, food, and exercise mandates can be like taking a newly sober person to their favorite bar, asking them not to drink, and then being shocked that they are having a miserable time. In the beginning, all your loved one might want to do is mess with their food and/or exercise, meaning to get back to their eating disorder!

As you reflect here, please be gentle with yourself for anything you didn't know prior to now. With this new wisdom, you have choices.

If you are wondering if something you're doing might be impacting your child and their eating disorder, it's a good time to stop, reassess, and have a conversation with them and your treatment provider(s) if you have them. You may also want to seek support or advice in a friends and family support group. (See chapter 1, **How do I find a support group?** section.)

What if I need to keep up my own food and exercise routines?

What does *need* mean to you? (We're not being snarky, we promise!)

We believe that when it comes to your own food and exercise routines, modeling flexibility is a remarkably supportive, influential thing you can do for your loved one. We all know the "Do as I say, not as I do" approach to parenting doesn't work well. That's especially true once a kid is old enough to have critical thinking skills.

Sometimes, a loved one's recovery process invites—even requires—parents and family members to change their own eating or exercise habits. Sometimes a parent finds that easy to do, and sometimes not.

Let's tease out need versus preference. See below:

- Alli rides her stationary bike to ease the pain in her arthritic knees. When she doesn't do it, they hurt more, which is more of a knee *need* than a preference.
- Jenny dances to express herself, and it provides her with a sense of community. She loves dance *so* much that in early recovery, she would eat an additional snack for every dance class her treatment team allowed her to take. While dance class isn't technically a survival *need* for her, it is one of many ways she fills her cup and is able to stay an energized live-in

recovery coach. Dance class is a very *strong* preference and possibly a need for her own sense of wholeness.

- If you have celiac disease, for example, eliminating gluten is absolutely a need.
- We've known people to be in the habit of using fat-free items only to discover that those were neither a need nor a preference—just a habit from their own childhoods or ideas about health.

Make sense?

It tends to help when, for the most part, you can eat whenever and whatever the person struggling to recover eats. Then they're not alone, and you are showing them the food isn't something to fear. But that's only within reason, of course. For instance, if your child is hypermetabolic and has a very large meal plan, we wouldn't expect a parent who is not also malnourished to replicate it.

In conclusion, if the need to keep up your own food and exercise routines is rooted in diet culture (e.g., favoring thin as the ultimate of health), healthism (pursuing health and wellness as a moral imperative), or disordered eating, please consider getting your own support.

When can I return to exercising or eating as I like?

Oh, you mean you're considering how your own practices may help or hinder your loved one's healing? If so, yay! That can be challenging to do. Major props to you. Our answer is this: It depends on how much your practices impact your child's path to wellness and healing.

We want to acknowledge that during a child's recovery period, a parent's food and exercise routines may be disrupted. Sometimes their bodies change. They may feel uncomfortable in their skin or miss their clothes that fit, etc. We've seen these experiences confuse even the most dedicated parents.

If this happens (or happened) to you, know that you are not alone. Regarding getting back to your own eating and exercise routines, here are ways to potentially navigate the path that can support all players. First, please consider what it would be like for your loved one—where they are in their vulnerabilities and recovery. Don't judge yourself about any of it! Instead, explore your thoughts and feelings about your body and eating with someone who will understand. That might be a partner, friend, religious advisor, support group, or someone else you trust. Better yet, another caregiver with personal experience, a provider who is trained in eating disorders, or a treatment team member may also help while offering an extra layer of understanding and empathy.

Jenny shares how she stays grounded when she is fully immersed in the life and eating routines of someone in early recovery:

> When doing live-in work, it is rare that I get to eat and move in ways that feel entirely organic to me. I have to be really flexible and strike a balance between taking care of myself and doing what's best for the recovery coaching clients I work with. I don't mean to equate my job with parenting; as I understand, they are not the same. Still, I can empathize with the challenges of having to deviate from one's schedule and preferences. This is why during live-ins, I prioritize sleeping at least eight hours, waking up early enough to meditate, keeping up with my social support circles, and making time to see my own therapist. Between live-ins, time off is imperative for my well-being.

Parents, you will probably need time off too. When you find yourself yearning to go back to the ways you were with food and movement prior to your child's diagnosis, that could be your cue to pass the baton to someone else and step away if you can—even if it's for a single meal, a walk with a friend, or an act of self-care. Hopefully, that action will alleviate at least some of the pull to return to old ways that could communicate confusing messages to your child or risk derailing their progress.

We can imagine this whole process of recovery feels challenging and asks so much of you at times. Wherever you are and whatever you *can* do, your loved one is undoubtedly benefiting from your efforts.

How do I know if I have a disordered relationship with food or exercise?

That can be tough to determine when our society is laden with healthism (preoccupation with personal health) and diet culture (slimness viewed as an ultimate ideal). We're going to give you a couple of tools to help you gauge your relationship to food, body, and exercise.

Many people who develop eating disorders—let alone disordered eating—have no idea they have gotten sick. Instead, they frequently think they need to find the "right" program or diet. Or they believe they're failing at dieting, exercising, or a health-promising food plan and must "just try harder." If you happen to discover you might be in trouble, please be gentle with yourself and seek support. Moving forward, you can help protect your child's recovery by adopting new practices and values.

The following is from Alli's book, *MeaningFULL: 23 Life-Changing Stories of Conquering Dieting, Weight, & Body Image Issues*:

> PEOPLE WHO STRUGGLE with eating and body issues often have practices and attitudes that span from slightly to severely disruptive to their lives. What's the difference between someone who's "always on a diet" and has body dislike versus someone with a clinical eating disorder? It depends. Here's a quick and easy generalization that might help you to conceptualize: a person with an eating disorder seems unable to "normally" eat. Their ***choices*** about food and exercise become "***I have to***" or "***I must***"; they cannot ***not*** do what they feel they need to do.[17]

Feel free to play with the above concept to see if you might be struggling yourself. Let's say that you prefer your salad dressing on the side. Challenge yourself: Order the salad already tossed—dressing *in* it. If you *cannot* eat it without freaking out, there may be a problem. Same with "If I have a bite, I'm afraid I'll eat the whole thing"-type beliefs. Take the bite. See what happens and notice your thoughts. Regarding your exercise, can you miss a workout without obsessing about it? Alli likes to say, "Do experiments and collect data." Both can be informative.

Another tool that might reveal if you could have a disordered relationship with food comes from Jenny's training: The Conscious Eating Assessment.[18] It's an informal, self-reflection tool, and a low-ish score may point to patterns worth noticing. We invite you to try it! Conscious eating can be a stepping stone along the way to the freedom of intuitive eating.

Conscious Eating Assessment[19]

Rate yourself on the questions below using a scale of 1 (you do not follow the guideline) to 10 (you do follow the guideline all the time). Track your answers on a separate paper and then total your score.

1. I'm conscious of my hunger. I eat when I'm hungry and don't purposely wait until I am starving.
2. I eat regularly and do not purposely skip meals or snacks.
3. I allow myself to eat all foods and don't exclude food out of fear. (This does not include foods you are allergic to or can't eat due to a diagnosed health condition.)
4. I eat what I want while taking into account nutrition information, such as getting enough protein or calories.
5. Even though some foods have greater nutritional value than others and are [viewed as] "healthier," I recognize that all calories are equal when it comes to gaining weight and that no certain food can make me gain weight, but certain eating habits can.
6. For most meals, I eat a balance of protein, fat, and carbohydrates.
7. I am conscious of when I am full and satisfied, and for the most part do not overeat past this point.
8. If I do overeat (which is normal to do sometimes), I don't make myself compensate for it or beat myself up, but accept it as a natural human thing to do from time to time.
9. I enjoy food and the pleasure of eating.
10. I make conscious choices to avoid foods or amounts that make me physically feel bad or ill after eating them.

Your total Conscious Eating Assessment score breakdown:

1–20 = A score in this range indicates that you likely have a distorted, unhealthy, and severely compromised relationship with food.

21–40 = A score in this range indicates that your relationship with food is likely problematic.

41–60 = A score in this range indicates that your relationship with food is likely out of balance.

61–80 = A score in this range indicates that there are likely areas needing attention, but you are already a somewhat Conscious Eater.

81–100 = A score in this range indicates that you are likely a Conscious Eater.

No need to stress about the score—it's not a judgment, just insight. The more you understand your own relationship with eating and body image, the more you can help your child heal.

Jenny would like to announce the following: "Not to brag, but my score landed somewhere in the nineties. I am a 'conscious' eater. In my eating disorder, I would have scored a fourteen, meaning I was a 'severely compromised' eater." The message is this: Parents, it can improve!

What if I don't want my kid eating "junk food"?

We cannot tell you how many parents have talked about feeling upset about seeing their children eating what they consider "junk food." Yet, for healing to happen, a kid may need to eat foods or quantities of food that can make a parent uncomfortable.

Commonly, the eventual goal of eating disorder recovery is intuitive eating, an anti-dieting approach that utilizes a person's internal wisdom. To explain a bit about why it can be vital for your loved one to eat what you consider junk food, we reached out to one of the foremost experts in this topic: Elyse Resch, MS, RDN, CEDS-C, Fiaedp, FADA, FAND, and co-author of *Intuitive Eating*.[20] She shares the following:

> Remember, this food is a source of energy and pleasure. If you attempt to regulate the amount of these foods, children will develop a sense that there are off-limit foods or foods that they can only eat occasionally or in small amounts. This makes these foods especially glamorous and exciting. Children will end up fearing that they won't be able to access these foods freely, and the fear of future deprivation might arise. Beyond that, a child with a

healthy ego is even likely to have rebellious feelings, because their autonomy is not being honored. A common result of deprivation and an attempt to control can be sneak eating when parents or roommates aren't home and bingeing on forbidden foods when they have free access, possibly at a friend's house, when they get to college, or once they have financial independence.

Rather than teaching them how to eat, we must help them eat in a way that creates trust in their intuitive wisdom about eating. I like to think of all foods as emotionally equivalent. Sure, some foods have more nutrient density than others, but all foods offer energy, and, we hope, most offer satisfaction. We don't want to teach our children to feel good about themselves for eating vegetables and bad about themselves for wanting cookies. No moral value should ever be attached to food choices.[21]

The ten principles of *Intuitive Eating* are below, and you can probably see how they can aid in recovery and freedom from an eating disorder:[22]

1. Reject Diet Culture
2. Honor Your Hunger
3. Make Peace with Food
4. Discover the Satisfaction Factor
5. Feel Your Fullness
6. Challenge the Food Police
7. Cope with Your Emotions with Kindness
8. Respect Your Body
9. Movement—Feel the Difference
10. Honor Your Health—Gentle Nutrition.

If you'd like to learn more about Intuitive Eating, Elyse Resch has authored and co-authored numerous books, which cater to different needs and ages: *Intuitive Eating* (the original, updated publication that's packed with the most science and research); *The Intuitive Eating Workbook*; *The Intuitive Eating Workbook for Teens*; *The Intuitive Eating Journal: Your Guided Journey for Nourishing a Healthy Relationship with Food*; and *The Intuitive Eating Card Deck: 50 Bite-Sized Ways to Make Peace with Food*.[23] Insider's tip: Intuitive eating is not the only approach people use to support healing from eating disorders, but you'll notice that many programs and providers utilize it.

If you want support with nutrition or feel you've lost self-trust about food and how to feed your kid with an eating disorder, you might benefit from the highly visual book that numerous parents have referenced throughout the years, *How to Nourish Your Child Through an Eating Disorder: A Simple, Plate-by-Plate Approach® to Rebuilding a Healthy Relationship with Food*, by Casey Crosbie, RD, CSSD, and Wendy Sterling, MS, RD, CSSD:[24]

> The Plate-by-Plate Approach® was designed to aid in the treatment of eating disorders, across all diagnoses, without measuring, counting, or numbers. The approach can be used alongside Family-Based Treatment as well as other treatment modalities. It is customizable to meet individual nutrition needs. It guides individuals and families to plate full and cohesive plates, while challenging the eating disorder with exposure and variety.[25]

In conclusion, stepping away from labeling food (e.g., "junk," "superfood," etc.) in a manner that ascribes magical powers or morality is the goal. To heal, your child may need to consume all foods without having a panic attack or meltdown, or feeling compelled to use compensatory behaviors, such as exercising, purging, and restricting.

4

Preparing for Treatment

Gearing up for treatment can feel daunting. This chapter covers information that can assist you in considering and then choosing which paths might benefit your child and family most.

Can we treat eating disorders like any addiction?

This question is, has been, and probably will continue to be highly controversial. Therefore, we consulted with Michael Lutter, MD, PhD, and author of *Gifted: Genetic Information for Treating Eating Disorders.*[1] Since 2007, Dr. Lutter, a physician-scientist, has used translational neuroscience approaches to improve the treatment of patients with depression, anxiety, and eating disorders. He clarifies the following:

> At first, it might seem like it makes sense to treat an eating disorder similar to how you treat addiction to drugs or alcohol, as both involve compulsive behaviors that can be difficult to stop engaging

in. The first major difference is that you need food to live, unlike, for example, gambling or cocaine. Because food is essential for survival, the body has multiple systems dedicated to ensuring that you eat the right amounts of food to meet your nutritional needs.

Recently, there has been speculation that ultra-processed or highly palatable foods may disrupt the body's normal self-regulation, leading to "addiction-like" behaviors.[2] Pop culture and even research tend to highlight dopamine as the culprit—a "fix." However, we don't have a clear idea of what causes "pleasure."

Contrary to popular belief, dopamine is not really a "pleasure" neurotransmitter. A better way to think about it is that it regulates reward valence (whether something is good or bad) and errors in the prediction of anticipated reward. So, what dopamine really tells you is if something is "much much better" or "much much worse" than your brain was anticipating. (Now does it make more sense about how music can "light up the brain" in ways that are similar to how cocaine or sugar does?)[3]

At this time, there are no clear answers about if food—even "sugary" or "highly palatable" foods—can be considered addictive in a traditional sense.[4] Consistent with this uncertainty, the *Diagnostic and Statistical Manual of Mental Disorders, Fifth Edition, Text Revision (DSM-5-TR)* does not classify eating disorders as addictions.[5] Also, there are currently no studies finding that treating eating disorders like addiction leads to better outcomes.

Still, some providers and treatment facilities will advertise that they treat eating disorders through an addiction model, or they believe in food addiction. If either means eliminating foods, please keep the following in mind: Research shows that intermittent access to a food—let alone attempting abstinence from it—can trigger cravings, preoccupations with, and bingeing on that food.[6]

From the perspective of this book, and as practical guidance for families, if your goal is for your loved one to eat without food exerting power over them, ask how the center or provider handles nutrition. What is their training background? What is their approach and eventual goal with clients? *How* do they guide clients toward that goal?

Some advertising keywords that might be helpful are *weight-inclusive, weight-neutral, anti-diet, non-diet, all-foods-fit*, and *Intuitive Eating*. Even so, we've all probably discovered (the hard way) that marketing can be very different than what's practiced. We encourage you to ask questions.

What are the levels of care?

Levels of care refer to a setting in which a person may receive treatment and that ideally matches their illness's severity, symptom frequency and duration, and need for support (psychological, medical, and nutritional). The options range from outpatient to inpatient. Below, we briefly explain each level of care (in order of least to most intensive) and highlight how your schedule and daily routines could be affected.

Outpatient

At this level of care, treatment can take place in a clinic that is attached to a hospital or larger treatment center or in individual clinicians' offices. The patient returns to their residence after their session(s) or program concludes for the day.

Outpatient treatment: A reference to outpatient can refer to both the various levels of outpatient care *and* to the least intensive level of care. For example, a client might be seen in a private practice. Therapist and dietitian appointments typically happen once or twice a week. Medical doctor and/or psychiatrist appointments occur on an as-recommended basis. Session frequencies and durations will vary among providers, but, for example, a typical therapy session is often around forty-five to fifty minutes. There could be more recommendations and appointments, but the rest of your life is likely business as usual regarding schedule.

Intensive outpatient programs (IOP): These commonly meet three to five hours a day, three to seven days a week. Each day might include snack time(s) and a group meal. Depending on the program, the snacks(s) and meal(s) may need to be packed at home, or they may be supplied for your loved one. IOP generally includes group therapy, family therapy, and individual therapy. Medical and psychiatric management are typically not included in the programming but may be required, meaning you'll have to ensure that your loved one has the necessary providers for this care.

Partial hospitalization programs (PHP): These can run approximately five to twelve hours a day, five to seven days a week. Most snacks and meals occur during treatment. Depending on the program, the snacks(s) and meal(s) may need to be packed at home, or they may be supplied for your loved one. PHP generally includes group therapy, family therapy, and individual therapy. The medical consultation offered may be limited. Psychiatric and nutritional management are usually incorporated in the programming. This level of care may also be called day treatment.

Finally, the term *day program* can refer to *PHP* or *IOP*.[7] If a provider refers to that, you might need to clarify which they mean.

Residential

Many people confuse or conflate residential treatment with inpatient care.[8] That's probably because it's around-the-clock care. There are significant differences: Residential treatment often occurs in a non-hospital setting, tends to have longer stays than inpatient hospitalizations, and is considered more intensive than outpatient but less so than the inpatient hospitalization level of care.

Residential treatment: People sometimes conversationally refer to this as "res," and it is when the person lives in a treatment setting—usually a home-like one. Generally, all meals occur there or on organized group meal outings and are typically supported and supervised by qualified program staff. Depending on the program, a client may obtain clearance to go out with you or independently while on a pass. The need for and intensity of medical and psychiatric attention are less than at an inpatient hospital level. Residential treatment centers generally include group therapy, family therapy, and individual therapy, along with psychiatric and nutritional management.

Inpatient

This level of care involves staying in a hospital or medical facility full-time and is the most intensive of the levels.

Inpatient hospitalization: Oftentimes shortened to "inpatient," this treatment level might occur due to a psychiatric or medical crisis, personal safety risk, or when residential care is not supportive enough. The structure of treatment will likely depend on whether the hospitalization is on a general psychiatric unit, a specialty eating disorder unit, or a general medical floor. Tube feeding might happen in this level of care. Inpatient hospital stays are not usually intended to be longterm but to manage or stabilize crisis and acute symptoms.

Inpatient psychiatric treatment for an eating disorder ideally takes place in a specialty eating disorders unit. There, providers should be well-informed about the medical and psychiatric needs of these conditions. However, you may not find a specialty eating disorders unit at your hospital, and your loved one may be treated on a general psychiatric unit. In either setting, programming can vary regarding whether any therapy is offered. Psychiatric management is typically included. Nutritional oversight for eating disorders will be provided in a specialty unit but might not be in a general one.

Inpatient hospitalization can also refer to an acute medical hospitalization. In the event that your loved one has critical medical needs, they will probably be treated on a general medical floor for the purposes of medical stabilization. Hopefully, providers caring for your loved one in this setting will be trained and informed about eating disorders and their treatment, but this is not always the case. Presently, there are some specialized eating disorder programs in the United States that handle acute medical stabilization specifically and cater to adults, minors, or both.

Please be aware that the details and labels for the above levels of care can vary. If you've been reading up on them or seeking treatment programs, you may have already noticed that. You'll probably benefit by clarifying what a professional or program states. For example, if a provider recommends "inpatient," it could mean anything from residential to acute medical stabilization.

The levels of care named in this section are the most customary categories.[9] If you feel somewhat unclear and want more detailed information, as the descriptions can seem confusing even to some professionals, watch the National Center of Excellence for Eating Disorders' "Demystifying Higher Levels of Care for Eating Disorders" on YouTube. Although it's geared toward clinicians, it provides an understanding and overview of the levels of care that you might find helpful.[10]

Viable, newer at-home options exist nowadays, too:

- Virtual treatment has become an option in this post-COVID-19 pandemic world. Each level (outpatient, IOP, and PHP) offers varying degrees of flexibility schedule-wise, depending on the program.

- Recovery coaching has emerged as a nonclinical, supportive adjunct to treatment, particularly when paired with outpatient levels and times of transition (e.g., discharging from a higher level of care, such as residential). When it comes to the schedule, coaching allows for flexibility. The day-to-day of live-in support is highly individualized and typically coordinated with the clinical team.

If your child is a minor, you should be included in some meetings at any level of care. (Yes, we said "should.") If your child is an adult *and* you are financially supporting them, paying for the treatment, or the treatment is on your insurance, it can be reasonable to be involved—even if that's in a limited way due to their legal rights as an adult.

Who are the members of an outpatient treatment team?

The composition of a treatment team can vary depending on the type of treatment your child receives. The typical clinical members include a therapist, dietitian, psychiatrist (or other psychiatric medication prescriber such as a nurse practitioner or physician assistant), and a primary care provider. (Because of cost or availability, a full team isn't always possible; focus on collaboration and the best mix of guidance you can find.) Brief overviews of these team members' roles follow:

- A therapist helps your child to better understand, manage, and heal the psychological pieces of this disorder along with other underlying issues and co-occurring disorders, such as anxiety, mood, substance use, etc.

- A dietitian focuses on the nutrition piece of care, which can include challenging food rules, supporting nutrition rehabilitation, and more. Note: "Nutritionist" is a broader term that may include individuals with and without formal training, so it can be wise to ask about their training and experience.
- A psychiatrist (or sometimes a psychiatric nurse practitioner or physician assistant) typically prescribes and manages psychotropic (brain) medications when needed. Some may also provide therapy.
- A medical doctor (or sometimes a nurse practitioner or physician assistant) monitors the physical risks and manifestations of the eating disorder.

Formal treatment guidelines generally recommend that treatment professionals cover the areas the eating disorder affects—mental, medical, and nutritional (see above). However, that might not apply to *all* approaches. For example, family-based treatment (FBT) sometimes does not utilize a dietitian. You'll benefit from understanding the standard practices and why various team members are or are not being recommended as healing progresses.

Providers we've seen added to the team, on a case-by-case basis, have included a somatic experiencing practitioner (SEP), case manager, other medical providers (e.g., gastroenterologist, cardiologist, endocrinologist), personal trainer, physical therapist, dentist, and of course, Jenny's favorite: recovery coaches.

Though not considered a typical team member, recovery coaches are becoming a more common nonclinical support addition. A recovery coach assists with the practical, day-to-day aspects of recovery, such as meal support, grocery shopping, exercise monitoring, etc., helping clients execute the treatment goals set by the clinical team.

What kinds of treatments are there?

Many approaches to treating eating disorders exist and are used in the various levels of care. They range from evidence-based (scientifically tested and with strong research support) to approaches commonly utilized or supported by some research, to adjunctive and non-Western modalities like yoga, reiki, and acupuncture, to in-person or online options. Let's take a closer look at these below.

Approaches and Treatments

At this time, the main nonpharmacological (non-drug) evidence-based treatments recommended in the United States include family-based treatment (FBT) and eating-disorder-focused cognitive behavioral therapy (CBT-ED), of which the most researched version is cognitive behavioral therapy enhanced (CBT-E).[11] They're considered frontline care per the *American Psychiatric Association Practice Guideline for the Treatment of Patients with Eating Disorders.*

FBT is the leading evidence-based treatment for an adolescent with anorexia nervosa.[12] FBT is a three-stage treatment consisting of around twenty sessions and lasting about a year. Stages include (1) full parental control and supervision of eating and related behaviors, (2) a gradual return of control to the adolescent, and (3) the adolescent establishing age-appropriate autonomy. Reported recovery rates for FBT range between thirty-five to about fifty percent at the end of treament.[13] Research suggests that if weight gain is required, a lack of weight gain by week four predicts that FBT is unlikely to be successful.[14] Should you choose the path of FBT, you will likely need to seek out a provider well-trained or certified in FBT. (If a practitioner advertises FBT-*informed*, you'll benefit by finding out, in detail, what that means before jumping in.) There are two popular books that could be helpful if you desire to better understand or utilize FBT: *Help Your Teenager Beat an Eating Disorder* by James Lock, MD, PhD, and Daniel Le Grange, PhD, and *When Your Teen Has an Eating Disorder: Practical Strategies to Help Your Teen Recover from Anorexia, Bulimia, and Binge Eating* by Lauren Muhlheim, PsyD, FAED, CEDS-C.[15]

CBT-ED is a time-limited treatment that has been tested in adults with anorexia nervosa, bulimia nervosa, and binge-eating disorder. It's recognized as a transdiagnostic (across diagnoses) treatment for eating disorders, and thus, it probably suits other specified feeding or eating disorder (OSFED), too.[16] CBT-ED consists typically of an assessment followed by twenty sessions, intended to take place over the course of twenty weeks (can be longer when weight restoration is needed).[17] The treatment includes keeping food records, establishing a regular eating schedule, and conducting behavioral experiments, all while addressing the thoughts, emotions, and cognitions that accompany each. Success rates seem to be about two-thirds.[18] Early behavioral change in CBT (e.g., more consistent eating, reductions in purging) predicts a favorable outcome.[19]

To comment on these modalities, we reached out to Lauren Muhlheim, PsyD, FAED, CEDS-C, who is a recognized expert in both. She shares, "Research has not revealed any specific factors in terms of family characteristics that predict successful treatment with FBT, so I believe that any family that is willing to do the work should be given the opportunity to support their teen at home." She also points out that some forms of CBT for eating disorders have been problematic regarding weight bias and for perpetuating weight stigma. She and her colleagues have published a new workbook to address that called *The Weight-Inclusive CBT Workbook for Eating Disorders: Tools to Reject Diet Culture, Heal Body Shame, and Promote Recovery*.[20] Lastly, Dr. Muhlheim highlights that "the great thing about both evidence-based treatments—FBT and CBT for eating disorders—is that you will know within one to two months whether progress is being made, and if it is not, you can pivot at that point to something else."[21]

If those approaches don't feel like a fit for you or your situation, have already been tried, or are not available to you, there are various other approaches commonly utilized by professionals to help people heal—some of which are considered evidence-based or emerging in their research support for eating disorders. The names or common acronyms and a tidbit, in layman's terms, about each follow (in alphabetical order):

- ACT—acceptance and commitment therapy is a process-oriented therapy that focuses on dealing with what feels hard or difficult via more acceptance and increased psychological flexibility, all anchored in personal, core values.[22]
- CBT—cognitive behavioral therapy is a well-researched talk therapy that focuses on challenging and then changing distorted, unhelpful thoughts and behaviors into more rational, helpful ones.[23]
  - Models of CBT for avoidant/restrictive food intake disorder (ARFID), such as CBT-AR, are being studied as emerging treatments.[24]
- DBT—dialectical behavior therapy is a therapy that combines mindfulness and behavioral techniques. DBT aims to teach people skills to manage intense emotions and improve one's ability for healthy coping and positive relationships. This modality is known for its compassionate applicability to supporting those with borderline personality disorder, high-risk suicidality, and many other mental health problems and disorders.[25]

- EMDR—eye movement desensitization and reprocessing is a structured therapy that uses protocols and procedures designed to help people reduce their distress connected to traumatic memories. Bilateral stimulation (alternating sensory stimuli that activate both sides of the brain) is a major component of this trauma treatment.[26]
- ERP—exposure and response prevention is a treatment that aims to reduce or build tolerance for anxiety through systematic exposures to triggers. ERP caters to elements of obsessive-compulsive disorder (OCD) and eating disorders.[27]
- FBT for bulimia nervosa in teens—please revisit starting at the third paragraph of this section.
- FBT for young adults—please revisit starting at the third paragraph of this section.
- ICAT—integrative cognitive affective therapy is a structured, short-term treatment that is emotion-focused and addresses behaviors associated with bulimia.[28]
- IFS—internal family systems is a non-pathologizing therapy that views the self as composed of many parts and sub-personalities and aims to heal the protective and wounded parts so the *Self* (the compassionate, calm, curious, connected parts) can lead.[29]
- IPT—interpersonal therapy is a time-limited, manualized treatment that focuses on how relationships affect mental health and improving both.[30] Throughout the years, IPT has often been compared to CBT-E regarding results, and it is recommended in the *Practice Guideline for the Treatment of Patients with Eating Disorders* for binge-eating disorder as an alternative to CBT-ED.[31]

- Psychodynamic therapy is a talk therapy (based on psychoanalysis—think Freud and the couch) that explores a person's past to increase insight about and self-awareness of their present motivations, conscious and unconscious.[32]
- Psychopharmacological (medicine/drug) interventions include medications such as fluoxetine for bulimia nervosa in adults.[33]
- RO-DBT—radically open-dialectical behavior therapy is different from the DBT that addresses impulsivity and undercontrol; this therapy uses, for example, mindfulness and skills training specifically to target overcontrol and problematic rigidity.[34]
- SE—somatic experiencing is a body-oriented therapeutic approach that focuses on understanding and changing the body's sensations linked to a traumatic event.[35]
- Trauma-informed therapies (those that incorporate the impact of trauma) may be more important than previously thought, as emerging data supports that trauma seems to play into eating disorder treatment outcomes.[36] Trauma is a person's psychological *response* to a distressing life event.[37] There's big *T* (e.g., war, rape) and little *t* trauma (e.g., everyday distressing events),[38] but trauma is a subjective experience. Many are walking around with trauma stored in their memories and bodies.[39]

This list is obviously not exhaustive. If something was left out, it doesn't necessarily mean anything negative. There are too many emerging and existing approaches to name.

Keep in mind, some commonly used healing modalities are harder to research or can't be replicated easily. Also, generally, the funding for eating disorders research in the United States has been low. Thus, scientific information is likely limited.[40] Furthermore, a lot of what we've learned from research came from mostly uniform participant pools, such as white and female.[41] Many factors can affect well-researched recommendations versus what's happening and helpful in clinical practice. The field is increasingly seeking and developing ways to address contemporary needs and better serve diverse backgrounds.[42]

Adjunctive and Non-Western Modalities

Less mainstream treatments may also be beneficial to some, such as acupuncture and reiki. Heck, one alternative approach that was considered unconventional as an eating disorders adjunct treatment has become common practice: yoga.[43] Chelsea Roff, an eating disorders researcher and the founder and director of Eat Breathe Thrive, a nonprofit working to prevent eating disorders and help people recover through yoga,[44] shares a bit of the history:

> For many years, cognitive-behavioural approaches have been considered the gold standard for treating eating disorders. But increasingly, researchers are recognizing that recovering from eating disorders is an embodied experience. It requires active engagement with food, our bodies, and other people. This is where yoga can help so much—yoga gives us an opportunity to practice noticing and responding to the body's needs, coping adaptively with emotion, and appreciating it for the life it allows us to live rather than what it looks like.[45]

The future of modalities and adjuncts is unknown, though it's safe to assume the field will keep evolving. Of course, your loved one is precious to you. With any approaches to healing, please ask your questions so you can be thoughtful about what might benefit your loved one, your family, and you the most.

In-Person Versus Online Treatment

That brings us to online versus in-person work. Since the COVID-19 pandemic began, there has been a rise in virtual treatment options, which has been extraordinary in many ways. Treatment can now be available to those in regions where no local help has existed. For individuals with autism or other sensory issues, virtual treatment might be preferred (or needed) and thus increases the number of viable treatment alternatives. People with chronic illnesses and mobility challenges now have more accessible options to receive help. For marginalized populations, such as transgender and gender expansive people as well as Black, Indigenous, and people of color (BIPOC), virtual treatment has opened more options to be with peers. Finally, people who can't or won't go to an office due to anxiety, schedule, commute issues, or other reasons can still receive help because of the addition of online support.

We both work online and in person. Though research supports that online eating disorder treatment can be quite effective,[46] we have experienced some limitations or trade-offs when using telemedicine options. Jenny points out the following regarding online recovery coaching: "During meal supervision—that's when I eat with clients, helping them to meet their meal plan or face a fear food—it's a lot harder for a client to hide food in person than it is on camera. It's also a lot harder for me to accurately gauge someone's portion sizes from a screen than it is in real life." Alli notes that during online therapy sessions, "Important nonverbal communication can be missed, like someone picking at their fingernails or shaking their leg. The screen doesn't show either. Subtle appearance changes (e.g., weight and skin-vibrancy) can easily go unnoticed until they're more drastic. And, when not in the same room, it can be easier for someone to disengage or even hang up on a provider." We share these examples for your awareness and consideration.

While we value that virtual treatment is an option for many, there is a different magic that happens when physically in the same room.[47] Anecdotally, a significant part of that magic has to do with energy, intuition, empathy, understanding, and connection. Even though these are possible virtually, we find that for us, there seems to be an amplifying effect when in person. We realize that sometimes it's not feasible to meet in the same room, but if it is, we encourage you to take advantage.

What is the best treatment?

There are so many factors that make something "the best." Yes, the quality of the provider and their training matter. Yes, the approach matters. Yes, the therapeutic alliance (the relationship between the therapist—or any provider for that matter—and client) usually matters to the outcome.[48] No, there is no one-size-fits-all: Someone else's "the best" doesn't necessarily mean that it will work for you and your family.

As you look for *your* best options and approaches, please keep the following in mind. If starting with an outpatient provider, which is where many begin, search for someone who is a specialist in knowledge and areas of eating disorders treatment. Important: "Specialist" is not a protected term; *any* individual can call themselves an eating disorders specialist or even an expert, so you'll probably need to vet the provider and their approach. How? Ask questions. Don't be shy about the screening process. Here are some ideas:

- What's their training in eating disorders and body image?
- What's their approach to treatment, and why?
- How do they evaluate if treatment is working?
- Do they believe people can be recovered?
- Are they a member of any eating disorders organizations, and if so, are they active in them?
- How long have they been treating eating disorders?
- What percent of their practice is typically focused on eating disorders?
- Are they affirming of the intersecting identities your child holds, such as neurodivergent-affirming, LGBTQIA+-affirming, etc.?
- What's the most recent eating disorders-specific conference or training they've attended?
- What do they see as the role and involvement of the parent(s) and other family members in the journey?
- Will they coordinate with other providers? How so? (For example, team communication can be beneficial when moving up or down in levels of care. Rather than the new team starting from scratch, the prior team can support, fill in blanks, point out known areas of struggle and triumph, etc.)
- Do they take insurance? Offer superbills only (a receipt for you to submit to insurance for potential out-of-network reimbursement)? Offer no superbill?

If anyone or anything (e.g., a facility, practice, nonprofit, book, etc.) implies a guarantee of success, be careful. Marketing pitches and promises can be hard to resist, especially during a crisis. Also, keep in mind that the most expensive doesn't necessarily mean "the best." Focus on a clinician's or program's specialization, experience, reputation, and vibe, which may or may not correlate with the cost of service.

When it comes to working with providers who have lived (personal) experience of eating disorders like us, that can be a valuable asset but isn't required. We know of many phenomenal professionals who have no eating disorder history. If having a provider with personal recovery experience is important to you or your loved one, you might want to ask the questions below as part of the screening process:

- Do they have lived experience of an eating disorder?
- Do they currently struggle with their own eating disorder?
- Do they consider themself to be recovered or in recovery, and what does that mean to them?
- If the answer is yes to any of the above, how does their lived experience inform how they work with clients with eating disorders?

Some providers may disclose in varying detail, and others not. But if you don't ask, you could miss helpful information.

To further aid in the screening process, the National Eating Disorders Association (NEDA) offers "Questions to Ask Treatment Providers," which is available online.[49] Also, when possible (and especially if you get a funky feeling), it's good to verify the status of a practitioner's credential or license to ensure they're in good standing. Professional licenses are regulated by state boards (such as the state medical board, state board of psychology, etc.). "Verify a license" is typically an option on state board websites; public disciplinary actions, if any, usually show up there. For recovery coaches, you might be able to confirm certification or training through the issuing organization (for example, the Carolyn Costin Institute) or ask for a reference.

Insider's tip: Some providers are willing to schedule a short consultation call at no charge. For instance, Jenny offers a free twenty-minute phone call or video meeting to prospective clients to decide if working together feels like it will be a good fit. Since there is no *guarantee* of success in mental health healing, it's important that both parties have hope and belief in a positive outcome (achieving healing goals), and the fit between parties matters. For example, Jenny says this to potential recovery coaching clients: "Can you imagine yourself being able to come to me in your most vulnerable moments?" For those who aren't appropriate for recovery coaching (e.g., they may benefit from more intensive treatment first), she offers them some guidance for the next steps. Therapists and dietitians sometimes manage inquiries similarly.

What do all the letters after people's names stand for?

First and foremost, "ED" does NOT stand for erectile dysfunction in our field! That said, the alphabet soup comes up often. We've grouped some of the abbreviations you may see when searching for providers. Treatment approaches and modalities would be covered here, too, (e.g., CBT, FBT, ACT, DBT, etc.), but you can find those earlier in this chapter. (See the **What kinds of treatment are there?** section.)

Usually, professionals will include some combination of academic degree, license, or certification(s) with their names or in advertisements (occasionally all, depending on the norms of the profession and state laws/regulations). In some cases, licensure, degrees, certifications, and/or credentials have shared letters. Below, we address (in alphabetical order) some of the abbreviations that you see with medical providers, nutrition providers, therapy providers, eating disorders recovery coaches, and eating disorders specialist certifications:

Medical Providers

Doctor: Academic degree

- DO—Doctor of Osteopathic Medicine
- MD—Doctor of Medicine

License or credential

- DO—doctor of osteopathic medicine
- MD—doctor of medicine

In the United States, there are significantly more doctors of medicine (MDs) than doctors of osteopathic medicine (DOs).[50] Both are licensed physicians who we typically visit when we see our doctor. MDs follow an allopathic (Western medicine) model, whereas DOs emphasize a holistic approach.

Nurse practitioner: Academic degree

- DNP—Doctor of Nursing Practice
- MSN—Master of Science in Nursing

License or credential

- APRN—advanced practice registered nurse
- NP—nurse practitioner
- RN—registered nurse

Depending on the state, a nurse practitioner (NP) may be able to prescribe certain medications. Sometimes, a psychiatric mental health nurse practitioner (PMHNP) can be a fit for psychotropic medication management in lieu of a psychiatrist. That is, assuming they have experience in treating eating disorders and take a collaborative approach.

Physician assistant: Academic degree

- MPAS—Master of Physician Assistant Studies
- MSPAS—Master of Science in Physician Assistant Studies

License or credential

- PA—physician assistant
- PA-C—physician assistant-certified

A physician assistant (PA) is a medical professional who is licensed to practice medicine under the supervision of a physician; they are not independently licensed.[51] A PA might offer an accessible option if an MD or DO is not readily available.

Nutrition Providers

Dietitians and Certified Nutritionists: Academic degree

- BS—Bachelor of Science (e.g., nutrition and dietetics)
- MS—Master of Science (same as above)

License or credential

- CNS—certified nutrition specialist
- RD—registered dietitian
- RDN—registered dietitian nutritionist

Regarding the RD and RDN, both titles are essentially the same thing. We must warn you about the following: In various states, anyone can hang a shingle out as a *nutritionist*. Without the CNS, RD, or RDN attached, the nutritionist may or may not have formal training.

Therapy Providers

Practitioners who can provide therapy include some medical personnel (depending on their training) and many licensed therapists, counselors, social workers, and psychologists.

Counselor, therapist, or social worker: Academic degree

- MA—Master of Arts (e.g., clinical mental health counseling, counseling, marriage and family therapy, or social work)
- MS—Master of Science (same as above)
- MSW—Master of Social Work

License or credential

- LMFT—licensed marriage and family therapist
- LMHC—licensed mental health counselor
- LPC—licensed professional counselor
- LCSW—licensed clinical social worker

Variations of the above licenses exist. For example, Alli has a second license titled licensed professional clinical counselor (LPCC). For social workers, there are quite a few titles, including licensed independent social worker (LISW) and licensed independent clinical social worker (LICSW). Further, licensed and pre-licensed designations can vary further by state. The *L* frequently indicates a licensed status. In California, though, an *A* can indicate an associate, which is a pre-licensed clinician (e.g., ASW and AMFT), which used to be an *I* for Intern instead. Hopefully, a provider's licensure information is clear in any listings or advertisements.

Psychologist: Academic degree

- PhD—Doctor of Philosophy (e.g., clinical psychology or counseling psychology)
- PsyD—Doctor of Psychology (same as above)

License or credential

- LP—licensed psychologist

A psychologist will likely have either degree's initials after their name and may or may not list LP. In addition to providing therapy, psychologists may also offer psychological testing and assessment.

Eating Disorder Recovery Coaches

Academic degree

- None required

License or credential

- None required (coaching is unregulated)
- CCIEDC—Carolyn Costin Institute eating disorder coach (the certification Jenny earned)

More coaching titles are out there. However, there are no national or state-regulated requirements for coaches. In other words, anyone can label and market themself as a recovery coach, eating disorder coach, or another kind of coach. We discuss possible screening questions in detail later in this chapter. (See the **What kind of training do coaches have?** section.) If you are considering bringing one on, you may want to ask providers and other parents for the names of coaches they recommend or trust.

Eating Disorders Specialist Certifications

At this moment, the only nationally recognized multidisciplinary certification specifically for eating disorders follows:

- CEDS—certified eating disorders specialist

If a C follows like this, CEDS-C, it means that the provider is also a CEDS-approved consultant. This credential has historically been administered by the International Association of Eating Disorders Professionals (IAEDP).

There are various specialist certifications and designations out there. There are also many bona fide eating disorders specialists and experts with no specialist credentials after their names.

There's no way to make the above list comprehensive. Alli served on an IAEDP committee that dealt with worldwide licenses and credentials: "I found the variations in just the United States to be wildly confusing! So, parents, if you're puzzled, it's not you—it's the organization and evolution of all this stuff that can be difficult to track." If you can, talk with a professional, even if it's an intake or exploratory call, inquire away.

No question is a silly question with any of these abbreviations (and in general). Save yourself time searching for answers online that may or may not make sense to you. A human, on the phone or in an email, can usually cut to the chase and provide the answers you need. Insider tip: Their response will give you a sense of them as a provider.

Do I need to look for an eating disorders specialist?

Ideally, yes! And we also know of people who have recovered without specialized treatment. There are no absolutes, only recommendations and *likely* safest, best practices.

To meet the standard of care for eating disorders, all treatment team members need to share common knowledge about eating disorders.[52] As a specialist therapist, Alli understands some of the medical and nutritional aspects of eating disorders. The same concept of shared knowledge in addition to one's own discipline applies to the other providers on the team.

When considering nonspecialized help, the phrase, "You don't know what you don't know," comes to mind. To us, the less providers know about eating disorders, the more you may have to depend on luck and chance. Given that these disorders are complex, have a high mortality rate, and can come with negative physical consequences, luck and chance are not what you want to rely on.

What if I can't find someone with specialty training?

The experience of having trouble finding someone with specialty training can be fairly common in certain geographical areas. The United States is large, with some densely populated urban areas and some that are spread out and quite rural. As a result, the number and types of providers available in any given part of the country, or even within a single state, can vary significantly.

Still, there are options. You might see if the non-specialist therapist or dietitian can help you find a specialist or if they can consult with one. Sometimes, without guidance, well-intentioned non-specialists may do more harm than good.[53] Other times, they can be helpful. If an eating disorders specialist isn't available, a combination of a non-specialist therapist with a skilled eating disorder recovery coach might be an option. Because recovery coaching is typically unregulated, many coaches are able to work virtually and legally across state lines. As we write this manuscript, there are moves to have more interstate licensure compacts (e.g., PSYPACT), which may open things up a bit by allowing providers, such as specialists, to practice across state lines.

We know from our own work of finding referrals in various states that sometimes the options are appallingly limited. Here's where fellow parents and support group members who have been there can be key. (See chapter 1, **How do I find a support group?** section.) Also, if you do find an expert located elsewhere, you can always ask if you can book a consultation or informational meeting to gather information and devise your plan. Seeing that specialist virtually may also be an option.

What kind of training do coaches have?

The eating disorders coaching industry is fairly new and not regulated. Anyone can call themself a coach, even without having any experience or education; whereas the credentials or licenses of other providers (e.g., dietitian, therapist) imply formal training and regulations. For your safety and quality of care, before bringing a coach onto the team, make sure they have gone through a certification or training process. While this is intended as a safeguard, it does not guarantee competence, particularly in an unregulated discipline—which is why we also provide some questions that might help you to decode a coach's level of experience.

Jenny recounts her training as a Carolyn Costin Institute (CCI) recovery coach:

> In addition to completing a rigorous twelve-module course that culminates in an internship with supervised coaching sessions, I'm obligated to complete continuing education units in order to keep my certificate current. The CCI curriculum was more rigorous than any course I took as an undergraduate at the University of California Berkeley or Antioch University.
>
> I also have a community of other CCI recovery coaches. We work collaboratively, bouncing ideas off one another, which is a way to expand knowledge and increase the quality of support. When I feel stuck about how to help a recovery coaching client reach their next treatment goal, I get supervision from an internationally acclaimed eating disorders expert, Carolyn Costin. As a CCI recovery coach, I'm held to high ethical and professional standards.
>
> I can't speak to the training of other eating disorders-related coaching programs. However, I hope my overview helps to share how much can be involved in becoming a competent eating disorder recovery coach.

Attention! If personal experience is the sole or main training of a coach, please beware: That is typically more of a peer mentor.

Despite the relative newness of recovery coaching, there are agencies that place coaches with clients. (This might work akin to a home help or employment agency.) Some of those coaches may be certified or trained, but there's not a guarantee—and as already mentioned, currently, there are no regulatory bodies like there are for other healthcare credentials, which means there is little to no legal recourse. We cannot stress the following enough: You'll need to ask questions. The following can be valuable during consultation calls:

- What training do they have? Any certifications?
- How long have they been coaching?
- Do they have past clients or parents of clients that would be willing to talk about their experience of working with a coach?
- Do they offer support between sessions? If so, what is that (e.g., text, phone, etc.), and do they charge a fee for that?
- If they have a specialty (ages, genders, diagnoses), what is that and why?
- What services do they offer (e.g., virtual, in-person, live-in, meal support, etc.)?
- How often do they typically communicate with the team?
- Who else do we need on the treatment team for coaching to be most effective?
- How often will they communicate with parents?
- What kinds of tools do they use for meal plan accountability (e.g., recovery apps, photos, meal support, texting)?
- Do they complete continuing education? If so, how often?
- Do they participate in any consultation groups for quality of care?
- What's an example of a difficult case, and how did they handle it?

If your child is struggling with a particular meal, snack, or time of day, you'll want to check that the coach is available to do sessions and/or text support during those time(s).

If adding a recovery coach to the care team, we hope the above helps you to identify a coach who is a great fit for your child and contributes to their (and your family's) healing.

Should I assemble the treatment team myself?

That depends. It can be strongest to hire one provider and have them assemble the recommended team for you, or ask them for referrals to other providers that they have worked with before. In either scenario, the team will likely share philosophies and approaches.

Here's why it's important for professionals—no matter how few or many—to communicate with each other and believe in the same or similar treatment philosophies. Let's say the dietitian believes in putting the parent one hundred percent in charge of cooking and feeding. The therapist believes in the client's autonomy and puts them one hundred percent in charge. Then, maybe the psychiatrist advocates that all parties collaborate and work together. Lack of treatment team cohesion leads to confusion and is often a space for the eating disorder to thrive.

This phenomenon shows up in parenting frequently. Here's a common example:

Kid: Mom, can I go to the movies?
Mom: No. (Kid goes to Dad.)
Kid: Dad, can I go to the movies?
Dad: Sure! Have fun.

Get the picture? It is so helpful if your child's team is aligned for treatment to be effective. Also, providers may be able to match up team members they believe will work well with your child, trust as professionals, and have established positive working relationships with. All in all, it is probably in your and your child's best interest to ask the provider you are speaking with (or plan to work with) if they prefer to guide you through building a cohesive team.

Is there a "best" insurance for eating disorders?

This comes up often—whether you don't have insurance and are shopping for it, have insurance and are wondering what it covers, or have insurance and are in a position to switch and/or obtain supplemental insurance.

To answer this, we contacted Dr. Rachel Presskreischer, an assistant professor in the Department of Psychiatry at the University of North Carolina, Chapel Hill. She has a PhD in Health and Public Policy and a Master of Science in Social Work. Her research focuses on access to treatment for people with mental health conditions. Below, Dr. Presskreischer offers guidance regarding insurance.

Unfortunately, there is no single answer to what is the "best" insurance plan when you or a family member has an eating disorder. Health insurance can be confusing and feel overwhelming—below are five general considerations to hopefully help.

1. What type of insurance do you (or your loved one) have?
People get their health insurance from different places including their employer, a state or federal health insurance exchange, or a government-funded plan of either Medicaid or Medicare. There are a lot of different health insurance companies, and some of them manage employer-sponsored plans, some manage government plans, and some manage both. If you have a plan through your employer, you'll want to clarify if it is a self-insured plan or a fully-insured plan. Different types of plans are required to comply with different laws and are regulated by different government agencies. Having this information can help you navigate any questions you have about coverage you are entitled to and who can help if you have any questions or concerns. *Health Insurance Basics* released by the Department of Health and Human Services, Department of Labor, and the Department of the Treasury

is a document that can help you understand your coverage and resolve billing problems.[54]

2. Does my plan cover intensive outpatient, partial hospitalization, residential, and/or inpatient levels of treatment?
Most plans, whether they are private or public/government sponsored, provide coverage for intensive outpatient and inpatient treatment. Other levels of care will vary depending on the plan. Additionally, make sure to check whether you are required to obtain prior authorization for any or all of these levels of care.

3. Does my plan offer coverage for nutrition services?
Coverage for nutrition services is highly variable, with some plans completely covering services and others not providing any coverage at all. One factor in determining coverage can be whether a particular state credentials and regulates nutritionists/dietitians. Without licensure, insurers may consider providers ineligible to bill for services, which may be particularly relevant for Medicaid. Medicare currently does not provide coverage for nutrition services for eating disorders.

If coverage is provided for nutrition services, it is useful to inquire as to whether there are certain services or diagnoses that are required in order for services to be covered.

4. Do I have coverage for out-of-network services? If yes, what is my financial responsibility?

a. Out-of-network benefits are offered in many private insurance plans and allow you to use a provider who does not accept your insurance plan and be reimbursed for all or a portion of the provider's fee.
b. If you have these benefits, you'll want to understand how much of the fee you are responsible for (after the deductible). If your plan says that they pay seventy percent out-of-network and you pay thirty percent, this is typically of an allowed or maximum amount that they pay for a particular service. As a result, this does not mean they will necessarily pay seventy percent of whatever the provider charges. If a provider's fee is $200 but the insurer's "allowed amount" is $150, they will pay seventy percent of $150 ($105), and you will

be responsible for the remaining forty-five dollars plus fifty dollars to get to the total $200 fee.

c. The process for submitting out-of-network claims varies depending on your insurer. However, all will likely require you to either directly submit or to include the information in what is called a superbill. Your provider should know what this means if you request one, but if not, what you'll need are

   1. date(s) of service
   2. provider's fee
   3. diagnosis code(s) (as a current ICD [International Classification of Diseases] code)
   4. procedure code(s) (typically called a CPT [Current Procedural Terminology] code)
   5. provider's first and last name
   6. provider's tax-id number
   7. provider's NPI (National Provider Identifier) number
   8. provider's contact information.

5. Can I access an advocate, case manager, or navigator through my insurer? Some insurance companies have an advocate or navigator service for enrollees that is there to offer support and guidance on benefits and resources to access. They can do things like assist in locating an in-network provider, help navigate the submission of claims, and answer questions about treatment options. This resource is typically different from just the person who answers the phone when you call the insurance number directly. There's no guarantee that this resource will be able to address all problems, but they may be an additional help in navigating treatment and benefits.[55]

Here are some resources for benefits and coverage information and assistance:

- your plan documents (which are required to be provided to you by your insurer)
- the human resources benefits coordinator at your employer
- an employee assistance program if your employer offers one

- marketplace insurance navigators (most states have these to help people navigate their options on the state marketplace)
- Project HEAL's insurance resource hub is loaded with helpful information, and their insurance navigation guides include links to information about letters and appeals processes, Medicaid eligibility, and Out2Enroll for LGBTQ+ people.[56]

And finally, since insurance can prohibit or grant access to treatment for many, here are a few more thoughts:

- Call and ask which insurances a particular treatment center or provider accepts if you or your child want to work with them.
- Check if a local specialist accepts insurance and which kind of insurance—some do.
- Talk to other caregivers about their experiences. There's a lot of creativity and solutions others have uncovered. Parents and caregivers can be powerfully resourceful, and they're often happy to share their own lessons. (See chapter 1, **How do I find a support group?** section.)

What should I know from a medical standpoint if my child is seen outpatient?

This answer is complicated and highly individual. Thus, it is beyond the scope of this book. For general medical guidance, we reached out to Jennifer Gaudiani, MD, CEDS-C, FAED, and author of *Sick Enough: A Guide to the Medical Complications of Eating Disorders and Undernutrition*.[57] Dr. Gaudiani shares what you can expect medically when/as your child stops bingeing, purging, and/or restricting:

Stopping Bingeing

When your child stops bingeing, usually it will be because they've embraced (or at least accepted) consistent, satisfying food throughout the day. Physically, they are likely to feel better, relieved of the achingly full post-binge states they were in before. In the absence of bingeing, some sleep better due to a less full stomach right before bed. Most redevelop physical hunger cues for the next meal or snack.

Stopping Purging

Stopping purging (typically by vomiting, laxative abuse, or diuretic abuse) is always a relief to the body, but it can get tricky medically.

Fluid shifts (rehydration and edema): Most people who purge are living life dehydrated, even if they drink plenty of fluids. That's because all three main methods of purging get rid of vital water and electrolytes from the body. So while individuals are purging, they may have a lower body weight. They could have a sense of a smaller body due to dehydration.

When they stop purging and hydrate appropriately, even if they are doing vital nutritional rehabilitation, their body appearance and weight might change overnight—a terrifying experience for many with eating disorders. This experience can be made less scary for them with good anticipatory education. For example

- Encourage good intake of fluids and electrolytes (these don't need to come in a packet; plain old-fashioned salty food will do!).
- Remind them how much better their muscles will work when hydrated and how they may feel less tired and headachy.
- Provide validation and compassion during this time.

Pseudo-Bartter Syndrome: Some people may develop a condition called pseudo-Bartter syndrome due to chronic dehydration from purging. Sometimes, but not always, it's indicated by a chronically elevated blood bicarbonate level. If that happens, a person's body might go past proper rehydration and actually retain fluids in their tissues, causing swollen feet, ankles, faces, and hands (edema). Wow is edema triggering. In rare cases, edema can be so severe that the heart, lungs, or brain are affected; this, of course, needs to be managed in a hospital setting.

People who have abused laxatives will likely experience the most severe and prolonged edema. Consult with your pediatrician/doctor before purging cessation (or if there's a history of edema with stopping purging). A couple of weeks of a low-dose prescription medicine called spironolactone might be needed. It is used for many conditions including acne and high blood pressure. Spironolactone blocks the hormone that causes that edema, and it can make purging cessation go more smoothly.

Painful, swollen cheeks: Some people who purge by vomiting and then stop can develop pain in their cheeks, ears, and throat. This can be accompanied by swelling near the angle of the jaw on both sides. This reflects temporary enlargement and inflammation of the parotid and salivary glands. Oftentimes sour candies, warm or cool compresses, and ibuprofen will help ease this over a week or two.

Severe constipation: People who have been abusing laxatives and stop may find it takes a while for their intestines to start working normally again. Usually, consistent food, proper hydration, and scheduled doses of gentle osmotic laxatives like polyethylene glycol (Miralax) will get things going again. When more support is needed, it's a good idea to call your pediatrician's/doctor's office.

Stopping Restricting

Stopping restricting usually means that your child is reintroducing appropriate food from the perspective of higher volume, variety, and caloric density.

Uncomfortable fullness, bloating, and even nausea: Most people who have restricted calories, *at any body weight*, will develop slowed stomach emptying (alongside slowed digestive function in general) called gastroparesis. When they start to eat enough again, they may feel painfully full in a way that lasts much longer than normal. Most often, this is extremely triggering, making meal and snack completion particularly challenging. However, it's those beautiful meals and snacks that will heal this over time as their metabolism speeds back up in the context of adequate nutrition!

Some people will need assistance via medications. Many others, however, will benefit from these two tips alone:

1. Liquids and semi-solids will digest faster than solids (and way faster than fruits, vegetables, and anything with high fiber).
2. Smaller volume meals that are more calorically dense may be scary from an emotional perspective, but they are way easier to manage digestively!

I like to give my patients the choice: "I know this is *so* uncomfortable, and it makes everything harder. You can choose to eat small portions of more caloric foods, or larger portions of 'safe' foods. What's non-negotiable is getting in all the nutrients your body needs!"

(Low) risk of refeeding syndrome: Historically, we thought we needed to start patients' calories out quite low as they stopped restricting, to prevent electrolyte shifts (especially of phosphorus) that can be quite dangerous if not medically monitored. However, study after study shows that yes, certain people need to start nutritional rehab in a medically monitored setting, but for the most part, even those people have a pretty low incidence of refeeding syndrome/low phosphorus levels. And we know now that the "underfeeding syndrome"—starting food intake too low and increasing too slowly—is probably more common and more dangerous than refeeding syndrome! When in doubt, ask a specialist.

Overall Recommendation

When it comes to stopping restriction, purging, and/or bingeing, my recommendation to parents is to follow their "spidey sense" regarding watching for medical issues. That is, *follow your intuition*. If you have a sense that your child isn't right, because they are acting differently, have meaningful new symptoms, or are expressing new fear or pain, listen to them and that sense and get them seen by a medical professional.[58]

What do all the treatment-related abbreviations mean?

As you move into treatment, you'll be communicating with providers who might use shorthand that's unfamiliar. Below is our version of a treatment-jargon translator, which includes popular acronyms and abbreviations that we freely utilize. You could encounter any of these when receiving or reviewing documents and correspondence. Select abbreviations appear below (in alphabetical order):

- AMA—against medical advice
- Bx—behaviors
- Ct—client
- Dx—diagnosis
- ED—eating disorder
- Hx—history
- LOC—level of care
  - Day tx—day treatment
  - IOP—intensive outpatient program
  - IP—inpatient
  - OP—outpatient
  - PHP—partial hospitalization program
  - PP—private practice
  - RTC—residential treatment center
- MNT—medical nutrition therapy
- Pt—patient
- RC—recovery coach
- ROI—release of information

- SH—self-harm
- SI—suicidal ideation
- SIB—self-injurious behaviors
- Sx—symptoms
- Tx—treatment
- WR—weight restored

5

About Treatment

Once a treatment path has been chosen, confusion inevitably arises. This chapter clarifies what to expect during treatment from the perspectives of insiders.

What is an authorization to exchange information?

An authorization to exchange information, which may also be referred to as a release of information (ROI) or a Health Insurance Portability and Accountability Act (HIPAA) release, is an important document. When signed, it grants permission for the center or provider to communicate with another person, professional, or entity about the individual with the eating disorder's treatment, wellness, status, progress, etc.

In our experience, it tends to be easier to get these permissions at the start when the therapy or recovery coaching client (adult or minor) is open versus after some time when they, or their eating disorder, may be feeling more closed off or defensive. Important initial releases include permission for

- all treatment team members to communicate with each other
- each team member to communicate with parents.

Those authorizations allow the opportunity for communication, as needed, so that your child's team and you can be on the same page.

The eating disorder sometimes makes people act in ways they wouldn't otherwise—like telling parents things to get a provider fired. Splitting is when people, such as providers and parents, receive different stories and might be played against each other either unintentionally or intentionally. Why would your loved one with an eating disorder do this? Sometimes, it's so they no longer have to participate in treatment.

In our respective roles, we notice a pattern: People who develop eating disorders tend to be smart and persuasive. When both of those are applied to splitting? Wow. It can make effective treatment nearly impossible. Splitting might look like a client telling a provider their parents said they have to scale back on sessions while telling their parents the provider said they don't need to meet as frequently, and neither are truthful. No, not everyone will do things to split, but just in case, we want you to know about it. Open communication, which a signed authorization typically allows, can be incredibly helpful to avoid splitting and facilitate consistent stories and messaging.

Finally, your child may be eighteen years old or over and say no to an ROI, or they have legal rights as a minor to exclude you from their treatment. Laws can vary by state. In these cases, you may simply have to accept that limit. However, if their argument to block you is that they're an adult or independent of you, *are they really*? If they are still dependent on you for school tuition, car insurance, health insurance, cell phone bills, housing, etc., that can highlight their continued dependence and open the door for a conversation about your involvement. Many parents have found it helpful to clarify that while they have legal rights to privacy, they are still financially dependent, and that continuing the financial support can come with conditions intended to ensure their safety.

Note: There are some exceptions to confidentiality; for example, if your child is at risk of suicide or serious harm to self or others, a release might not be required for a provider to communicate with a legal guardian or parent. With all the intricacies and assumptions around confidentiality for adults and minors, it's best to have a conversation with your child and provider to clarify the limits of privacy and confidentiality (e.g., what information can be shared with you and what legally must be shared with third parties, such as child or adult protective services, police, etc.).

How often should I be included in sessions or treatment?

The frequency depends on age, need, level of independence, the treatment facility or provider's policies, and more. If you are not being included in treatment, we invite you to ask your loved one, the provider, and the facility:

- Do they plan to include you? If not, why?
- Do they offer any family support or education groups, recommended readings, etc.?

Start a conversation. Share why participating is important to you. With eating disorders education, family and friends can often learn to be supportive and protective of healing.

If you are not being included in sessions or treatment, what about adding a family therapist as supplemental support? Family therapy can provide a space to facilitate communication within the family system, which includes the person with the eating disorder. What we're trying to get across is this: Some providers or treatment facilities won't ask you to participate. Perhaps that's because of their policy, their beliefs about autonomy, your child asking for you not to be included, or something else. Family therapy tends to take the focus off the identified patient (person with the illness) and allows any willing family members to be involved.

Finally, your child's response to treatment might prompt you to include yourself. Here's what we mean: If your loved one ends up in a residential or inpatient setting, you could receive communications (phone calls, texts, emails) begging you to bring them home or to stop treatment. Even in the best programs, some people will swear they are being tortured. Phrases such as, "They're trying to kill me," "The staff doesn't know what they're doing," "Everyone here is sicker than me," "Save your money; this isn't going to work," "They're not even making me eat" are some we have heard. These kinds of claims are probably the eating disorder making a desperate attempt to find a way out of treatment, but understandably, caring parents will want to verify that they're not based in truth. Getting to the bottom of the claims can take a lot of your time and energy, worry, etc. Sometimes, asking for a joint meeting with you, your loved one, and their treatment team to discuss what's going on may put a damper on splitting (presenting different narratives to you and their team) that's happening.

Bottom line: Your involvement may vary based on what's been mentioned above. We encourage you to take steps necessary to facilitate helpful communication with your child during the treatment process.

What indicates that my child needs a higher or lower level of care?

We've seen the following factors alone, or in combination, cause the provider(s) to consider moving a client up or down in levels of care:[1]

- medical status improves/declines or stabilizes/destabilizes
- safety with self (e.g., intensity, frequency, and severity of self-harm and level of suicidality) changes
- another simultaneously occurring disorder or diagnosis worsens/improves
- treatment responsiveness or lack of responsiveness
- motivation for change (recovery) strengthens or weakens
- willingness/unwillingness or ability/inability to try more healthy behaviors, actions, and thoughts
- eating disorder symptoms worsen or improve
- problematic behaviors decrease, increase, or stay the same
- other life-interfering behaviors arise
- need for increased or decreased support
- financial conditions change (e.g., insurance cuts off or approves a new level of care, which the client qualifies for, cash pay runs out, etc.)
- treatment compliance or noncompliance occurs (following or not following the treatment plan).

Ideally, your treatment team will guide your loved one's process. If you use your health coverage, which many people need to do, insurance will significantly impact your child's level of care.

Insider's tip: If you're feeling concerned that your child needs more support than an outpatient setting can provide, you or they might reach out to a treatment center for an assessment. That may help to inform you and your loved one.

What should I tell people if my child goes away for treatment?

We believe giving your child some input about what gets shared is often appropriate. What do they want you to tell other people? If they'd prefer you to be honest, great! That makes it easiest. But what if they want you to do something like lie or hide it? *Why* do they want you to do that? Maybe they're feeling ashamed, scared, or guilty, and that is valuable information. Their reason gives you insight into their emotional state. From there, you may be able to agree on something that works for you both.

To be clear, we aren't suggesting you lie for your loved one. That can create an awkward, uncomfortable situation, and this is already tough enough on you! So it may be important to find a veiled or vague response that respects their privacy but doesn't compromise your morals or values. A couple we have heard include "They're off doing some personal growth" and "They're doing a self-improvement program. I'll leave it up to them to share details."

For your own peace of mind and sense of safety, it's important to think about who you're sharing with, how they might respond, and whether they have the capacity to support you. Unfortunately, even well-meaning family members or friends don't always "get it" when they learn someone has, or is receiving treatment for, an eating disorder. Their reactions and advice can sometimes feel overly simplistic, isolating, unhelpful, unrealistic, or even shaming.

If that's happened to you, you're not alone. Remember that eating disorders are still widely misunderstood by the public.[2] Take your time. Go slowly and see if you feel supported before opening up more.

Lastly, make sure others directly involved (e.g., family members in the know) also understand what's appropriate to be shared, what's private, etc. This can be especially important due to social media because if someone posts something you or your child are not comfortable with, it's much harder to control the public narrative at that point.

Does my child need to be on medication?

When parents ask either of us this question, we direct them to a medical provider. Generally, therapists have limits as to how much and what they can say about medications due to scope of practice (what a professional license legally allows). And it would be inappropriate for recovery coaches to give medication advice.

Because psychiatrists specialize in this area, we reached out to an eating disorders expert, Vikas Duvvuri, MD, PhD, DFAPA. Dr. Duvvuri, a psychiatrist-neuroscientist trained at Caltech and Stanford, has helped start several eating disorders programs, including one at UC San Diego. Most recently, he founded Sunol Hills in the San Francisco Bay area to provide comprehensive care for eating disorders and mental health. Here's what he says:

> This question is the crux of many conversations with parents. However, it's typically wrapped into, "How do I get my child back (as nothing has worked so far)?" So, my answer is this: How about we do whatever it takes to get your child back?
>
> Sometimes, the conversation then moves to specifics and strategy around medication/med choices. We discuss what

symptoms or problems are most important to reduce for recovery. Examples follow:

- If eating disorder-related anxiety is very high despite environmental and behavioral approaches, then meds could make a big difference for some.
- If depression is a barrier that is not relenting, meds can often remove that roadblock and accelerate recovery.
- If the child has had trouble sleeping while sick, they often become resigned, accepting the idea that insomnia is here to stay. Helping restart good sleep patterns—which can be assisted by meds—can have an exceptionally large impact on anxiety reduction, mood, energy, and general level of function.

Both environmental approaches and meds are often needed for a reset.

It's important to be aware: If the adult/minor has lost a lot of weight and remains stuck, weight restoration needs to become a priority. A higher level of care may be necessary, and medication can be incorporated in that setting.

With some parents and people with eating disorders alike, fears around using meds surface: "Will they become dependent on meds?" "How long will they need to take meds?" "How can it be their recovery if they are using meds?" "One friend took a particular med and had this bad experience; I don't want that." "I'm afraid that meds will make me gain weight."

The role of meds is to reduce the barriers to recovery. Complex conditions like eating disorders can come with many comorbidities. Thus, med usage needs to be highly personalized, prioritizing the *most critical issues first.*

Research surveys show that those recovered from eating disorders are more often than not *no longer* on meds. This highlights the need to optimize med usage to successfully navigate the recovery process—but not necessarily forever. We want to limit the psychological and medical scars that could otherwise remain.[3]

When considering medications, it's best, if possible, to consult with a psychiatrist (nurse practitioner or physician's assistant) who specializes in eating disorders—or is at least eating disorders-informed. A professional who is knowledgeable about which medications tend to be most effective for people with eating disorders, which ones should and should not be used with a particular diagnosis or behavior, and how those medication choices could affect healing, will probably serve your child and you.

What if my child won't eat in front of me?

This can happen and usually needs attention during the healing process. We suggest asking your kid, teen, or adult child *why* they don't want to eat in front of you—of course, in a non-defensive way, like, "I'm curious. It appears that eating in front of me seems difficult for you. Can you help me understand what's going on?"

So much of figuring out how to help someone to recover is about collecting data to find the path that helps unlock their healing. For instance, Jenny had a recovery coaching client who wouldn't eat in front of her mother because the mom had a lot of her own food rules, and the kiddo had shame eating foods that Mom deemed "bad." So the team found others that the child would eat with.

If your loved one won't eat with you, they may truly be unable to do so right now. Is there someone they *will* eat in front of? A family friend? A teacher? Someone else who they can struggle through meals with, such as an online meal support group or a recovery coach? Is there a guidance counselor at school? All public educational facilities (kindergarten through grade twelve) in the United States that receive federal funding offer a Section 504 plan that allows for accommodations. If you're in a position where a 504 plan could benefit your child, "How to Tell the School of Your Child's Eating Disorder Needs," by Eva Musby, is an online resource that may serve you.[4]

Sometimes, the eating disorder is so strong that the person may promise to eat, but they can't on their own. Especially in early recovery, it's often helpful—even necessary at times—for meals to be overseen to ensure the prescribed meal plan is being met; providers refer to that as meal support or supervised meals. If your child won't eat in front of you, for now, that may not be a problem as long as they have someone they will eat with when they need support and accountability.

What if the team or my loved one is asking me to be less involved?

There are so many reasons why that might happen. For example, particularly in older treatment approaches, family and parents were often not included. A provider—or client themself—might have a bias against parental involvement. The child could be too emotionally activated by a parent, thus affecting progress. Whatever the reason, please think about what *you* believe could be most beneficial to your child's healing, and advocate for that.

Nowadays, many of us see parents and family as part of the treatment team. Caregivers can be huge assets and strengths. Having said that, there can also be instances when a parent's participation can become unhelpful. For instance, wanting improvement desperately, sometimes well-meaning parents can unintentionally sabotage progress by undermining goals and strategies set by the team. (Imagine a parent with limited medical background overseeing or directing a surgeon in an operating room.) Understandably, parents can have anxiety about progress, and sometimes they may hold unrealistic expectations. As an example, Jenny worked with a recovery coaching client whose parents wanted every meal and snack to be a challenge or fear food for them to get over the eating disorder more quickly. This client thought she was *failing* both treatment and her parents—when she was actually making progress! (We've seen this type of situation play out repeatedly.)

The prior scenario could easily cause the team to ask a parent to change course. Ideally, parents can trust the team's recommendations and collaborate regarding the child's treatment. And if there is confusion or disagreement, a talk with the provider or providers (if authorized) will likely be beneficial.

If you are feeling excluded from the process, keep asking questions and sharing that you want to be involved. Take it from there. Also, this may be an instance where seeking your own help might soften the rigid boundary keeping you out. (See chapter 1, **How do I find a support group?** section.)

Insider's tip: Keep in mind that nothing stops you from sharing what you observe or your concerns with a member of the treatment team. They may not be able to comment back due to confidentiality, but your observations can be vital. For example, sometimes your loved one's eating disorder is reporting "I didn't purge," "I haven't exercised this week," "I don't binge," or "I ate every meal and snack" to providers. Yet, let's say that you heard your loved one vomit, checked their location app—they were at the gym, noticed unauthorized food delivery charges, or found their meal and snack in the trash. Sharing what you witness or suspect can be so helpful! The therapist or treatment center may need to tell your loved one how they got the information. Even so, your sharing could be the golden ticket to change or progress. In our opinion, truth is one of the antidotes to this disorder.

What if I don't want to be involved in my child's treatment?

That is a parent's choice. Still, we believe it can pose a significant impediment, especially if the kid, teen, or adult with the eating disorder is still living in your home.

Jenny has worked with recovery coaching clients whose parents have told her they don't wish to participate in treatment for various reasons. (If you are reading this book, that's probably not you.) For those clients, Jenny encourages them to appreciate the support their parents *are* providing (e.g., by offering to pay for treatment). She then encourages them to actively lean on their team.

Sometimes, a parent keeps a distance because of the misperception that eating disorders are not *real* disorders. Other times, the parent is dealing with their own mental health issues or another life stressor such as divorce, a sick relative, another child with special needs, etc. Perhaps they weren't raised to acknowledge psychiatric illness. Any of those could stop a parent from participating in their child's treatment. In these cases, even if only one participates in the actual treatment, try to be on the same page. It's important that the primary caregivers—if there is more than one—are aligned in messaging, rules to help healing, etc. That consistency tends to be what is in your child's best interest.

Can my child continue to exercise during treatment?

It will probably be safest to ask the professionals overseeing your child's care for their guidance. If you don't have a team in place, then you may need to rely on your best judgment. Talk with your child;

express your concerns. It can be wise to err on the side of caution while your loved one's body is doing much-needed repair work in early recovery.

Getting out of a nutritional deficit accrued during an eating disorder can take time. Complications pertaining to energy availability, cardiovascular health, electrolytes, biomedical function markers, sex hormones, and body composition may have arisen during the eating disorder.[5] Any exercise can be dangerous if someone's body is stressed or medically compromised. Think about a car heading over a hill on fumes—it's a bad idea. Not only can it run out of gas, but what might it do to the car's engine and other parts?

On one hand, many treatment facilities and providers have had a policy of little to no exercise in early treatment. On the other hand, emerging research is showing that physical activity can offer potential benefits for people undergoing treatment for eating disorders.[6] Studies have shown it can reduce the compulsion to exercise, increase physical strength, enhance quality of life, and more; further, a published single case report indicates it might also repair cardiac abnormalities in those with anorexia nervosa.[7] As hopeful as all this sounds, proper oversight of physical activity is key. Safety is imperative, and exercise can be tricky as it's commonly a symptom of an eating disorder and can go to extremes, such as dysfunctional exercise.

Dysfunctional exercise (e.g., pushing past pain or exercising on an injury because one feels they *have to*, obsessing about calories the activity will burn, etc.) is known to precede, maintain, and exacerbate eating disorders.[8] So even if your child is consuming adequate nutrition and is not medically compromised, dysfunctional exercise does not support recovery.

Many in the eating disorders field emphasize movement where the purpose of activity shifts from weight control or punishment for eating to pleasure, self-expression, mental health, etc. Jenny shares an example of what her return to exercise looked like in early recovery:

> Dysfunctional exercise was a big part of my eating disorder, but before that, dance was a passion and my first love. Totally abstaining from exercise wouldn't have taught me how to differentiate self-destructive versus life-affirming movement, which would have been catastrophic upon discharge from treatment.
>
> While the exposure of going to a dance studio to take a class—and standing in front of the mirror—was a challenge, I'm eternally grateful I was afforded the opportunity to work through it with the support of my team and peers. Including supervised exercise as part of my treatment experience prepared me for a return to dance. Moreover, it allowed me to move again, not to punish myself, but to appreciate all the magnificent ways my body can express itself.
>
> I will always dance, and it will forever be a part of who I am.

As mentioned, Alli did her recovery in a different way and at a different time. She recalls

> When I first started dance class as a kid, I loved it. Then, during my decades of eating disorders, dance became mostly about body criticism and calorie burn. Once I began recovering, I stopped any exercise that had become a torment.
>
> Cut to years later: While meeting up with a friend, there's an open house happening next door at a dance-fitness studio. The owner invites us in. I discover it's super inclusive and not body focused. Everyone's sweating and smiling. (What?) I try it and rediscover something I value but had taken a very long break from. Not only do I enjoy the movement to music, but I also like

> the sense of community there. I become a regular at the weekly Broadway-style class.
>
> Then, during the pandemic, my beloved dance-fitness studio closed, and a teacher moved one class to a public park. For years now, I have been attending that class weekly with a bunch of lovable goofballs, a background of kids playing, and dogs on their evening walks. Finding a sense of satisfaction and community through dance unpaired it from any dysfunction.

Provided your child wants exercise in their life, making sure movement is integrated in a healthy and balanced way, rather than disordered, is imperative. Research has begun to break down the level of attention and care needed to approach exercise in a therapeutic manner. Literature suggests guidelines such as involving a team of trained professionals, assessing medical stability, inquiring about unhelpful exercise-related thoughts, setting boundaries and limitations around the way exercise will be executed, and taking a gradual and individualized approach.[9] It further highlights that when it comes to specific types of exercise, working on physical flexibility is often the safest way to start; resistance training supports restoring body mass, and cardio activities can be tricky as they have the potential to be misused by those with eating disorders. When possible, consulting with an experienced professional can pave the safest path.[10]

If your child's team recommends abstaining from exercise for a period of time, we would like to reassure you that it may be a *for now* but doesn't have to be a *forever*. However, if your loved one decides not to exercise at all, that's their choice and right, too. Our hope and belief is that they can someday return to the physical activities they once loved, if they want to, or perhaps discover new ones that bring satisfaction, joy, or connection for the very first time.

Can my child recover as a vegan or vegetarian?

It depends. For some, eating as a vegan or vegetarian can be rooted in a deeply held belief system, a commitment driven by a moral stance: This is commonly referred to as an ethical vegan or ethical vegetarian. For others, eating as a vegan or vegetarian may provide a socially acceptable label that allows them to limit and avoid foods. If it's the first, then recovery as a vegan or vegetarian is possible for some, and may benefit from guidance by a dietitian who understands and supports plant-based recovery (when accessible).

Deciphering which camp—ethical or eating disorder—your child falls in can be complicated. We reached out to an expert with professional and lived (personal) experience of eating disorders and veganism to shed some light on this. Jenn Friedman, a Licensed Mental Health Counselor and the author of *Veganism and Eating Disorder Recovery*,[11] shares her insights:

> Consider the following, which may help you to get a sense of whether they are truly an ethical vegan or ethical vegetarian.
>
> - Why did they become a vegan or vegetarian in the first place?
> - How have they reacted to discovering information about animal mistreatment in the past?
> - Where else do their vegan or vegetarian values show up in their lives? For example, if they are vegan, do they make an effort to avoid animal-derived clothing (e.g., wool, leather, etc.)?
>
> You could inquire:
>
> - How would you differentiate between an aversion to meat and dairy and an aversion to your fear foods (those they avoid due to the eating disorder)?
> - Does your idea of recovery include eating vegan or vegetarian versions of your fear foods (e.g., vegan ice cream)?

If you notice that the answers don't seem to be motivated by their ethics, then their food choices are likely serving their eating disorder. If that's the case, professional guidance that is catered to their specific recovery goals can support the introduction of non-vegan or non-vegetarian foods.

If they really are ethically vegan or ethically vegetarian, you can support them with solutions or alternatives to limitations they encounter. For example, maybe there is a vegan alternative that meets the same nutritional requirements as a non-vegan version. Maybe there is a high-protein vegan yogurt or mock-meat burger, etc. If you live far from a grocery store that contains plant-based substitutions, maybe there is a way to have these items delivered to your home.

However, there may be times that avoiding all animal products may be particularly difficult. The definition of veganism (which can be adapted to vegetarianism) is doing that which is "possible and practicable."[12] Ironically, just like the process of recovery, the practice of veganism is not about perfection, but rather, making conscientious efforts when feasible.[13]

Veganism and vegetarianism both put compassionate treatment of sentient beings (e.g., animals) at the forefront. And in many ways, you can use that to help challenge your loved one's eating disorder because isn't your child a sentient being, worthy of compassionate treatment too? "Would you make your pet vomit if they ate a treat?" "Would you purposely underfeed a pet?" That kind of questioning may infuriate your child's eating disorder but may also create some dissonance between their moral beliefs and the way the eating disorder makes a person think.

What should I expect after treatment?

Transitions can be difficult for many, and the transition after treatment is no exception. Hopefully, your child will be stable enough to start reintegrating into life *without* eating disorder behaviors. They may still have thoughts and urges, though. At best, they are in a place to navigate these without acting on them. At worst, they could have slips (when they use an eating disorder behavior without fully relapsing) or relapse. Most likely, you can expect something in between.

The recommended standard of care is a gradual step-down level of support, such as residential to partial hospitalization or intensive outpatient to outpatient (e.g., private practice).[14] Notice how each decreases in level of intensity. That is to enable your child to adjust to each reduction of support while growing in their self-reliance skills.

While moving from each level to the next, or out of treatment altogether, something called discharge planning is essential and includes various considerations: What's the next plan? What are the resources? What's the schedule going to be? Are facilities or providers secured so your loved one can step down without a gap in care? If there's going to be a lapse in care, how will you and your loved one manage that? Additionally, with limited financial or geographical resources, discharge planning might become a creative process of combining support groups with other available resources.

Ideally, your child's facility or provider leads the discharge planning process. However, that may not always happen (e.g., some don't do the planning, insurance abruptly cuts off covering program costs prematurely, etc.).

The goal is for clients to no longer need their providers someday because they have replaced them with their own dependable internal guidance, social support, and other resources (e.g., spirituality, hobbies, extracurriculars, etc.), but that can take time. Co-occurring disorders may still need psychological care. Growth and recovery needs may continue to warrant attention. Or life, coping, and social skills could use additional time to bloom. Some clients do best with maintaining ongoing support while building their next phases of life. For instance, a therapist, dietitian, or recovery coach (possibly all of them) may be optimal for a while, even if functioning mainly as a security blanket.

How soon can my loved one return to school, sports, their job, etc.?

That will depend on specifics—severity of disorder, progress, what the doctor says, what the team agrees on, what you think, what your loved one wants, school or athletic policies, and so much more. We understand that life has demands and deadlines. A yearning to get back to "normal," such as dinners and holidays without eating and mental health struggles, is completely understandable. Please be gentle with yourself if you experience impatience and frustration.

You know that saying, "Haste makes waste"? Rushing back to school, sports, their job, etc. often leads to crashing. Providers commonly recommend a gradual reintroduction, which could look like them taking less intense classes or returning to a sport recreationally prior to competitively, depending on medical stability and readiness. In some cases, educational accommodations may be key to your child's ultimate success. You want their recovery pace to be sustainable in the *long term*, right? If you find yourself wanting to push in a way that's too fast, take a deep breath and focus on longevity—recovery is often a marathon, not a sprint.

What if I don't think treatment is working?

If you are fortunate enough to have a team on board right now (and you have an authorization or permission), ask their thoughts about treatment goals and your loved one's progress and prognosis. Hopefully, that gives more clarity. If not, how long have you and your loved one tried to change the eating disorder-related thoughts, behaviors, and attitudes?

There are various ways to treat eating disorders, so if one doesn't work or only works a little, your loved one may need different treatment, more consistency, or simply more time. To get a sense of what's going on and where their process is, the following questions could be helpful to ask your loved one:

- How free of your eating disorder do you want to be?
- Do you think you are there?
- What's been helpful so far?
- Where are you feeling stuck?

Take in the information. Recognize that the eating disorder may be strong, and being under or malnourished can stall progress. If you feel unclear, reach out to people who are knowledgeable about eating disorders and discuss your thoughts, questions, and concerns.

If nothing seems to be moving toward wellness, it may be time to reassess the plan going forward. But before that, the following might be a helpful conceptualization of your child's healing journey. Are you familiar with the stages of change model—precontemplation, contemplation, preparation, action, maintenance, and termination—that people often use for addictions?[15] Below is Alli's interpretation of those stages of change, applied to eating disorders:

Precontemplation

In this stage, your loved one does not recognize their problem. If you address it, you may hear something like, "You're overreacting" or "Don't be ridiculous."

During *precontemplation*, educating yourself on eating disorders and expressing loving concern might be your strongest approach. When caregivers use scare tactics to jolt their loved ones into change

("You could *die*!"), it's often ineffective at convincing the person that something is wrong. Instead, being curious and gently noticing changes might help your loved one experience some beneficial self-awareness (e.g., "It seems like you don't spend as much time with your friends anymore. Anything you want to talk about?" or "I can't help but notice you're not eating what you bake for us").

To move to the next stage, *contemplation*, your loved one will need to overcome at least some of their lack of awareness or denial about their disorder. For example, they mentally tally enough negative or uncomfortable consequences to begin to believe there might be a problem (e.g., getting caught sneaking food, missing social events, or getting tired of constantly thinking about food).

Contemplation

In this stage, your loved one may somewhat acknowledge having an eating disorder. They might call it something less severe, such as "emotional eating" or "a little too much exercise." They may think something along the lines of, "It would probably be good if I fixed this, but . . ."

During *contemplation*, it may be particularly helpful for you to ask them process-oriented questions (those they cannot answer with a single word, yes, or no). "What's this like for you?" "How do you feel that it helps your life?" "How do you feel that it's not beneficial or hurts you?" If your loved one engages, it gives them opportunities to grapple with their potential dilemma and to increase their awareness.

To move to the next stage, *preparation,* your loved one will need a reason (or a few). Maybe the negative consequences of their eating disorder attitudes and behaviors grab their attention, they acquiesce to someone's concern about them, or something else moves them towards change.

Preparation

In this stage, your loved one is probably unsure of how or what to change. Still, they're trying to plan for it (e.g., reading about treatment, self-help articles). They may display a push and pull, such as a seemingly strong "I'm ready" to change (e.g., start therapy, stop purging, eat more), followed by an inability or refusal to do so.

During *preparation*, their age and level of independence will affect how you can best aid your loved one. Offering your support could be helpful (e.g., to locate qualified specialist therapists or treatment facilities).

To move to the next stage, *action*, your loved one will need to experience something internal, external, or both that pushes them to be open to more action than prepping and research. The impetus could be keeping a promise to someone (maybe you!), wanting something to be different regarding their disorder and its impact on their life, feeling deeply exhausted, etc.

Action

In this stage, the bulk of the work happens, and a lot can be frightening and difficult for your loved one. They're typically practicing abstaining from behaviors (or trying to), eating for nutritional rehabilitation, and working to change their eating disorder-related obsessions and compulsions. They may need to challenge and change long-held beliefs about self, others, food, exercise, and more. They face fears and often yearn for their old ways (also known as the eating disorder). Warning: A reduction in symptoms can be accompanied by an increase in distress—that means while they are getting better, they will likely feel worse! It is especially during this time that people might return to earlier stages.

During *action*, because your loved one is trying to meet so many challenges, validating their feelings could provide especially needed emotional uplift (e.g., "That sounds scary," and "I see how hard you are working"). Also, inquire about how you might support them. They may say "I don't know." That's OK; their task may be to start figuring that out.

To move to the next stage, *maintenance*, your loved one will need to practice and learn to trust the new beliefs, skills, and behaviors. As you can imagine, building that trust can take time, repetition, insight, and self-awareness.

Maintenance

In this stage, whatever healing has been established and practiced tends to deepen and become more routine. A shift from the *action* to the *maintenance* stage can seem indiscernible at first to both your loved one and to you; for example, sometimes, you might hear your loved one sounding or see them doing things similar to the action phase. At other times, they seem utterly solid in their non-eating disordered ways.

During *maintenance*, as a caregiver, you may not have much to do regarding the eating disorder. Your support will likely be needed or requested around life stressors not related to the eating disorder. It's *almost* as if you get to be a parent of a kid without an eating disorder.

To move to the next stage, *termination*, your loved one will need to keep practicing their skills, solidifying their healing.

Termination

This stage is full recovery, which is often possible over time. Your loved one may strive for this stage or slip into it due to repetition and practice. I have heard more than one recovered person say these types of statements: "I didn't realize I was fully recovered until the worst thing happened, and I had zero eating disordered thoughts or behaviors," or "I didn't even realize the eating disorder's absence until well after I had dealt with something horrible."

Circling back to earlier stages of change is quite natural anywhere along the way to *termination* (such a harsh title for a glorious phase!) Rest assured: Loopbacks—which can look like slips and relapses—cannot erase the healing skills and understandings already built, making a true back at square one implausible.

On a note of hope, in my experience, the circling back to earlier stages often builds solidity in eventual recovery. Think of it like when you forget something at the store: You circle back for the item. You don't have to re-shop for *everything*—just whatever was needed.

For additional reading, various resources detailing stages of change for eating disorders or phases of recovery are available. Most do not cater to caregivers. So, we want to highlight another that does. "Stages of Change," by the National Eating Disorders Collaboration, offers actions to consider taking with each stage.[16]

Insider's tip: It's challenging to notice the thinking or belief changes your loved one might be making until you *see* different behaviors. And yet, the internal work (e.g., thought and attitude shifts) is often forward movement and progress. Still, keep in mind that while waiting for readiness, time may be of the essence—a conundrum with these disorders.

How can I trust that a provider cares and isn't just taking my money?

We so understand this question! Who hasn't wondered? Jenny shares her point of view as a recovery coach and a person with recovery experience:

> In early recovery, my eating disorder fed me a lie that the people around me only cared because they were being paid. I know this is an all-too-common belief among those being treated for their eating disorders.
>
> Nowadays, I like to say what Carolyn Costin said to me that made a difference: "You pay me for my time. You don't pay me for my love. I choose to do that."
>
> I'm grateful to be in a position where I can keep in touch with my recovery coaching clients after we end our work together. When I'm out in the world and see something that reminds me of a client or family I've worked with, I often reach out and text them;

> they often do the same. This tether that remains, even after our work together is complete, is evidence that care and connection aren't transactional.

Alli explains her position:

> As a therapist, I have different rules than Jenny. For example, it's generally frowned upon to reach out to former clients once treatment has ended. Though I don't necessarily like all the rules and regulations placed on therapists, I also recognize that a therapist's ethical guidelines exist for good reasons.
>
> I believe that a provider's care shows up in how the professional speaks and listens to you. It's in the interactions. Hopefully, my clients sense it quickly. They still may argue about or question if I sincerely care about them, and I understand that. Yet with enough time, they'll feel it.
>
> This question brings me back to a moment in graduate school. I was learning about therapists being encouraged to have *unconditional positive regard* for our clients. I remember asking, "Isn't that love?" The professor gave me a vague, unsatisfying answer.
>
> Now that I'm around two decades and hundreds of clients into my journey as a therapist, I can tell you: It is care and love—with boundaries and rules that have to be honored—but it's authentic and real.

We can't tell you exactly *how* to trust that a provider genuinely cares and is not just taking your money. However, if you can observe that they are competent, want to help you, and care about doing a good job of helping you (e.g., they listen to you and have skills), that can be enough. In the end, we hope you will *feel* some sense of care and be able to trust yourself and them when it's present.

6

Obstacles to Healing

Complications on the road to recovery happen and can feel exasperating. This chapter bolsters your skill set so you can navigate your path with foresight and resolve, steering around potential obstacles.

What if we can't afford the recommended treatment?

We wish that everyone had access to the recommended care, regardless of finances. If you can't afford or don't have insurance that amply covers the optimal care for eating disorders, please don't lose hope. We provide you with some avenues to explore below.

Organizations

Carolyn Costin Institute (CCI) offers sessions—typically three to four hours—with recovery coaches in their internship phase for no fee. At the time of this writing, Carolyn Costin herself supervises the interns' work. Many certified recovery coaches, Jenny included, offer pro bono slots or work on a sliding scale for those with financial limitations.[1]

Eating Disorders Anonymous (EDA), a Twelve-Step fellowship, describes itself as individuals sharing their "experience, strength and hope with each other" so people "may solve their common problems and help others to recover from their eating disorders."[2] EDA offers no-cost support. The belief in full recovery and focus on balance, not abstinence, sets EDA apart from other food and eating-related twelve-step programs.

The National Alliance for Eating Disorders (The Alliance) tends to stay informed about lower-fee options and often helps individuals with unique needs and circumstances access treatment.[3]

National Association for Anorexia Nervosa and Associated Disorders (ANAD) describes itself as "the largest peer support resource for eating disorders in the country."[4] ANAD provides a wide variety of support groups for people with eating disorders and their loved ones.[5]

ANAD also offers a recovery mentor program: "free eating disorder support online for those who struggle with eating disorders but are motivated to recover. ANAD mentors are people who have walked the difficult road to recovery from their eating disorder and are recovered for at least two years. Mentors spend six months working with and supporting their mentees as a source of hope, wisdom, and empathy."[6]

Project HEAL (PH) offers Treatment Access support for eating disorders treatment, pairing individuals facing financial and systemic barriers to care with providers and treatment programs who offer sliding scale and pro bono services.[7] We're aware of PH beneficiaries who use PH's pro bono and sliding-scale services in conjunction with non-specialist providers who are sometimes covered by their insurances.

Solid recovery can be possible, even with financial constraints.

Medical Guidance

Eating disorders are psychological illnesses with medical consequences. Your child may be able to be seen by a doctor covered by your insurance. If that's not possible, some community agencies offer low-cost medical services. For support regarding the medical aspect of eating disorders, feel free to refer back to sections in earlier chapters that address this. (See chapter 1, **What's the first thing I should do if my loved one has an eating disorder?**, **Should my child go to a doctor immediately?** and **What if the doctor gives my child a clean bill of health?** sections. Also see chapter 4, **What should I know from a medical standpoint if my child is seen outpatient?** section.)

Self-Help

If your loved one is interested and motivated, various self-help books are available. Of note, the Centre for Clinical Interventions provides a workbook online, at no cost, titled *Break Free from ED (Eating Disorders).*[8]

People with eating disorders may seek guidance and comfort in recovery memoirs, as these books seem like a combination of inspiration and self-help. Warning: Recovery memoirs sometimes inspire and help the eating disorder! Many tend to focus heavily on the illness itself, which can be unhelpful or triggering for readers.[9] Alli shares her observations as a therapist:

> Over the years, quite a few clients have talked about how reading recovery memoirs inspired them to compete with the author's lowest weight, hours without food, worst eating disorder day details, etc. They also have used the book's details to directly

compare in ways that invalidate their own experience. I've heard justification like, "So-and-so did X, Y, and Z. So I'm not *that* bad."

When approached thoughtfully and with a clear balance between illness and wellness, memoirs have the potential to support. At the very least, they should avoid doing harm.[10] Yet there's currently no content warning or system in place to help readers know in advance whether a particular book might be distressing or risky to read.

Outpatient Sliding-Scale Psychological and Nutritional Treatment

Therapists who are in training to become eating disorder specialists might be a beneficial and more affordable option. Some of these clinicians work under the supervision of experienced, licensed professionals in private or group practices. Others offer services through community agencies and university mental health clinics, where therapy is often available on a low-fee or sliding-scale basis. Additionally, dietitians in private practice and group practices may offer affordable options. When contacting therapists and dietitians in particular, feel free to ask if they offer a sliding scale or if they provide anything at a lower fee.

Therapy, Nutrition, and Support Groups

There are many groups, tailored to specific needs, both online and in person. An eating disorders therapy, nutrition, or support group may be catered to a specific population (e.g., midlife, pregnancy, teens, or a particular diagnosis) or focused on a topic (e.g., eating disorders education, intuitive eating, or dietary challenges). Groups may provide cost-effective additional support or, when appropriate, an alternative to individual work.

Please note that people respond differently to group settings. For some, groups can unintentionally trigger competition or reinforce eating disorder behaviors, while for others, they become a place of healing and connection. Insider's tip: If they are willing, have your loved one try a few until one meets their needs. Encourage them to attend more than once before deciding whether it's a fit or not (unless they felt too disrupted, unsafe, or triggered).

Intensive Outpatient Treatment

If private practice and community agency providers aren't financially feasible, consider looking into in-network intensive outpatient programs (IOPs). If your loved one meets the criteria for this level of care, it might be covered by insurance. While it's not always a long-term solution, it can provide critical support in the short term.

Insurance and Employee Assistance Programs

If you have health insurance, you may want to check your provider directory for in-network eating disorder specialists. Some of the multidisciplinary team members might accept insurance. Additionally, an employee assistance program (EAP) can be a helpful resource for referrals.

You'll probably notice quickly that many of the specialized clinicians choose not to accept insurance. Factors such as low reimbursement rates or insurance restrictions on treatment duration likely contribute to why. The following blog post offers more information: "Having Trouble Finding an Eating Disorder Therapist Who Takes Insurance? Here's Why," by Lauren Muhlheim and Alli.[11]

There are many options to explore. The above are meant to spark ideas since supporting someone with an eating disorder can sometimes require creativity on everyone's part. You may want to ask others who have experience with eating disorders treatment how they have navigated it. A group brainstorming session can be key for understanding existing structures and creative problem-solving.

What if I don't want to upset my child or hurt their feelings?

Of course, you don't want to hurt your child's feelings! Nevertheless, it will likely help their recovery (and adulting) if you can be lovingly stronger than their eating disorder and willfulness. And yes, that may sometimes mean upsetting them.

Imagine babysitting a toddler. You're both playing in the front yard. You notice a car speeding down the street just as the toddler tries to run into the road. Would you reach out and hold the toddler back? Of course you would! And if the toddler kicked, screamed, and threw a tantrum, yelling, "I hate you!" would you release them and allow them to run into oncoming traffic? Of course not.

Sometimes, upsetting your child is in *their* best interest. And, when it comes to hard decisions regarding treatment, if you have a professional, a team, or a support group to discuss those with, that's probably going to be in *your* and your child's best interest. (See chapter 1, **How do I find a support group?** section.)

We've noticed a trend in our therapy and recovery coaching practices: People with eating disorders are often determined and influential. They usually know how to get their way, even outside of the eating disorder. Two examples follow:

1. A straight-A student wants to take extra units (credit hours over a full-time status). While you admire their drive, you are deeply concerned about their school-life balance.

2. Your child wants to hang out more with someone who you believe is a "bad" influence. Your gut says, "not a good idea," but you don't want to disappoint or alienate them.

If either of these sounds familiar, it might be time to start changing the pattern. You can still respect their autonomy and invite conversation while sticking to your beliefs about what's in their best interest. Consider these potential responses to the prior scenarios:

1. "Can you help me understand why you feel the need to take on more? I'm concerned that you rarely have any downtime."
2. "I know you really want to hang out with your friend, but I don't have a good feeling about it. Even though it might upset you, no."

Your child may not like being challenged, but they may benefit from you having created containment and structure. Jenny reflects on her journey: "I needed someone to not just look at the eating disorder but at the bigger picture of how I was living my life. The above examples of limits are something that I believe would have helped in my own recovery and perfectionism."

There can be some unexpected positives to your child becoming upset or saying they're hurt. Verbally expressing themself allows them to identify feelings, communicate, and grow in recovery. Instead of using food, bingeing, restricting, or compensatory behaviors to speak *for* them, they're using their voice to express their thoughts and feelings. So, yay! Also, if your kid has a strong reaction to your limits (as if *you* are in trouble with them), it does not necessarily mean you did something wrong. You may have done the best thing for them and their healing, and that can majorly upset the eating disorder part of them. A lot of parents grow to recognize when it's the disorder versus their loved one responding.

Warning: Verbal threats or physical violence cross the line and are not appropriate communication from them or you. Be careful of giving your loved one a pass for unacceptable behavior because "They're sick." For example, we've witnessed kids yell "shut up" and "f&*k you" at their parents. Food has been thrown *at* the caregivers—not just on the floor during a tantrum-like episode. It's important to communicate which behaviors are not acceptable to you.

We encourage you to address inappropriate behaviors in a timely, productive way. That may mean being direct, such as saying, "Not acceptable," "Stop," "That's rude!" or whatever resonates with your home's values. In addition to calling out the behavior, in some cases, you might consider a consequence to help them remember what's not OK. Why? If you don't say or do anything, you could be teaching your child how to treat friends, family, and romantic partners. Furthermore, if events are escalating into verbal or physical abuse, or if you are fearing for the safety of yourself, your loved one, or anyone in your home, you might contact emergency services (e.g., 911) or a mobile crisis team.

What if my partner/co-parent doesn't take this seriously?

First, we want to acknowledge how frustrating and hurtful this probably feels to you. Here's where a lack of a united front can cause problems, creating a setup for the eating disorder to thrive.

We address two situations below: parents living in the same household and parents living in separate households. In both scenarios, one parent does not seem to take the eating disorder as seriously as the other.

Parents Living in the Same Household

Imagine two executives in charge of the same office and equal in decision-making power. If they are in alignment (united in policies, decisions, values, etc.), the office probably runs relatively smoothly. Now imagine those bosses having different rules, expectations, deadlines, etc.

Employees amuck!

Parents in agreement is usually the strongest setup. If your partner or co-parent doesn't regard this disorder or treatment with the same reverence as you do, can they let you take the lead and echo your message in words and actions? Insider's tip: Consider answering your child with "Let me talk to your mother/father/my partner first." When you and your partner/co-parent follow through by getting on the same page before making decisions, the *feel* of a united front will likely be achieved.

Parents Living in Separate Households

Here's an experience that gave Jenny special insight about recovering while living in two homes. The parents were divorced and on two different pages about a lot of things. She shares:

> When I was traveling back and forth with my recovery coaching client, I noticed that each home was distinct in attitudes, beliefs, and approaches to daily life as well as recovery. My client seemed to chameleon (I'm using that as a verb to paint a picture), adapting to each environment. I even caught myself doing the same (e.g., abiding by unspoken rules, absorbing the household's energies and values). I could empathize a great deal.
>
> I kept sharing eating disorders education and setting boundaries. The kid kept showing up with noticeable changes. Between the

two, eventually, the home that had initially been less concerned about the eating disorder began to understand the effort and commitment required for their daughter to recover. They stepped up and grew, learning how to provide effective meal support and sit through tough conversations.

Sometimes, a provider talking to your co-parent or seeing the dedication your child is putting into recovery can be a game-changer. That was the case in this situation.

We share that example because it shows that people who weren't bought in can buy in.

If you don't have a Jenny or a provider, what about someone with personal experience of an eating disorder or another caregiver from your support group? Could they talk to your partner or co-parent? What about an informational meeting with a specialist? Alli has had parents and whole families attend a single consult (informational meeting where they can ask questions) with a goal of aligning with each other more.

If the partner absolutely cannot jump on board, the following may provide some semblance of unity, predictability, and consistency:

- having a unified treatment team
- creating the anchors in both homes—favorite foods (even if that means packing these for your child to bring to the other home), duplicate essentials such as toiletries, clothing, phone charger, etc.
- packing transitional objects like a favorite blanket and recovery journal that can be easily transported between both homes
- keeping the appointment schedule intact, no matter which home they are at.

Jenny has seen the above work in her live-in situations, which is another instance where recovery coaching can give helpful insight as to what is happening in the home.

While having one parent or partner who seems less committed to the recovery process can pose unique challenges in treatment, it doesn't have to be insurmountable. And if none of the above suggestions help to get your partner or co-parent to take your child's eating disorder seriously, this happens sometimes, and you are not alone.

Why might I need to "fire myself" from parenting?

We're not going to say "fire yourself" altogether. Instead, consider your child's current developmental needs.

We witness dedicated, loving parents and caregivers. They are often quick to solve problems for their kid(s). They're excellent at anticipating their loved one's wants and taking care of their needs. (If others have ever complimented your effectiveness, problem-solving skills, or similar qualities, this could be you!)

There comes a point in a child's development when they, particularly during the teenage or young adult years, may miss opportunities to cultivate their critical thinking skills and sense of self-efficacy. Why does this happen? Because their parents do so much for them. Alli sometimes tells parents they may be "too good" at their parenting skills (and she means it!): too efficient, resourceful, and organized for what's needed for their child's development. Additionally, to recover from eating disorders, individuals of any age often need to foster greater self-trust and agency. If this scenario could apply to your situation, here's something straightforward and immediately doable from Alli:

Get curious. For instance, before advising or solving something for your kid, *stop*. Ask your loved one, "What do you think?" "How might you solve this?" or "What are your ideas?" Then, wait.

Silence. That's right: Awkward! (If it seems called for, reassure them with something like "It's OK if you don't know. I'm interested in your thoughts.") Then try to wait for them to answer *before* offering your solutions or suggestions.

This approach will give you a lot of information about where they are in their critical thinking skills. Importantly, it will give them the opportunity to exercise and strengthen those skills.

Ideas to try: If you find it challenging to break the habit of fixing and offering solutions immediately, sometimes exhaling once or saying, "Let me think about that for a bit," can give them (and you) a beneficial pause—space for growth. Taking this a step further, you could encourage your loved one to try one to three things on their own before coming to/coming back to you for help. (Unless there's an emergency, of course.)

Regarding parenting and the eating disorder specifically, your level of involvement can feel confusing. Sometimes, you might need to shop for your loved one, cook for them, run out and get what they are willing to eat, let them miss school, make life easier, etc. Yet other times, that kind of accommodating stops your loved one's necessary growth. It can be challenging to tease out which is which and what is what. If you are privileged to have providers on the team, they should be able to offer guidance. If you don't have a team, please bring up this topic in a support group. You may get mixed feedback, but hopefully it helps. (See chapter 1, **How do I find a support group?** section.)

We understand that it can be tough to watch your loved one struggle. And here's the heart of the matter: If you do their homework for them, what's the result? There is no way they can learn what they need to know. They must do the work themselves to grasp the necessary lessons. Additionally, there is value in allowing your loved one to fail (yes, the other f-word) from time to time. Flailing and failing (within reason) grants them the opportunity to pick themselves back up again, which can build resilience and confidence in their ability to problem-solve.

How might having more than one diagnosis affect healing?

Having more than one diagnosis can complicate healing, but it's typically manageable.

Co-occurring disorders (sometimes referred to as comorbidities) are common among individuals with eating disorders.[12] A 2022 review article revealed the most prevalent: anxiety disorders, mood disorders, post-traumatic stress disorder, and substance use disorders. Others that followed included personality disorders, neurodevelopmental disorders, obsessive-compulsive disorder, non-suicidal self-injury (self-harm), and various physical illnesses.[13]

Psychiatric and medical disorders can emerge during the course of an eating disorder or precede it. Though another condition may be less immediately dangerous than an eating disorder, it may still impede progress. Diagnoses including but not limited to mood disorders, attention-deficit/hyperactivity disorder (ADHD), obsessive-compulsive disorder (OCD), and autism spectrum disorder (ASD) can impact motivation, interoceptive awareness (ability to understand the body's internal sensations and signals), and more, posing an additional obstacle to healing.

As a therapist, Alli has experienced this situation quite a few times. When she finds herself perplexed, "Why hasn't this worked by now?" or "Those are really good treatment programs; why didn't healing stick?", that's her cue to explore what else is keeping the eating disorder active. Even if a co-occurring issue is less dangerous than the eating disorder and usually would not need urgent attention, it might now. Thus, if a treatment isn't working, especially if that treatment has shown success in studies or you've given it a sufficient try, consider if there might be another diagnosis potentially in the way.

If you have a full team, the therapist, psychiatrist, or both typically address psychological co-occurring disorders. The medical provider usually leads the management of medical co-occurring disorders. Recovery coaches seek consultation from other team members or specialists who can guide them, or they may help the family find a specialist to treat the co-occurring issue.

Sometimes, supplemental psychological testing (standardized tests and assessments focused on psychological and behavioral characteristics) may be needed to clarify the clinical picture. In some cases, a formal psychological evaluation helps to confirm the presence or acuity of other mental health disorder(s) co-occurring with the eating disorder (e.g., ASD and personality disorders). That information can meaningfully inform treatment.

Does body image ever improve?

Yes, it can. Many people report that their body image seems to improve when they focus on appreciating the ways their body functions. As an example, for someone who can sit and stand, they can't deny that their thighs help them do that many times a day. Even if they hate the appearance of their thighs, their thighs are serving them. Also consider what they like to do: We're talking about horseback riding, dance, sports, listening to music, etc. Finding gratitude for the things one's body allows them to do often helps offset discomfort about how it looks or feels.[14] Further, body image can become less distressing when one's life is full of things they derive satisfaction from or enjoy—there's less room and time to be consumed with body-focused thoughts.

On the topic of body image, some terms that confuse folks follow: body positivity, body neutrality, and positive body image. Understanding the nuances of each can be important to overall critical thinking about your loved one's healing.

Body Positivity

Body positivity came from the Fat Rights Movement in the 1960s.[15] Social media seemingly co-opted the movement (e.g., #BoPo) and transformed it into what is typically seen today as body positivity: promoting body love and celebration of every size, texture, shape, fatness, perceived imperfection, etc.[16] For many, the current in-your-face portrayals of body positivity, particularly on social media, can seem discouraging, unattainable, or insincere. (We have even said so ourselves!) It makes sense that body neutrality discussions began appearing on social media and in clinical practices as an alternative.

Body Neutrality

Similar to what we described at the top of this section, body neutrality focuses less on appearance and more on recognizing what your body does for you that allows you to engage in life. It promotes taking a neutral stance on your body; that means not necessarily loving, liking, disliking, or hating, but caring for, appreciating, and respecting it. For many with body image issues, body neutrality can seem more attainable, and thus more pursuable, than the over-the-top version of body positivity. Body neutrality might be a stop on the way to positive body image.[17]

Positive Body Image

This broader, more holistic concept extends beyond the physical body to include the self inside the skin. Positive body image is multidimensional: It includes body appreciation, functionality appreciation, body compassion, a broad idea of beauty, body image that's flexible (e.g., accepting that we have bad body image days), and more.[18] Positive body image is not just a concept; it's a well-established academic field, offering research and insights into body image healing and self-acceptance.

If you notice that your child struggles with body image while other aspects of recovery improve, that's par for the course. When someone loathes their shape, size, or skin they are in, even disliking their body just a little less can take time. Alli reflects, "When I first started learning about eating disorders treatment, I kept hearing that body image is one of the last things to improve. That has held true anecdotally around two decades later."

Can my loved one live in this diet culture world and still get better?

Even without having met your loved one, we believe they can! Here's why: Many people recover despite the societal presence of diet culture (societal valuing of thinness) and healthism (making health into a moral value). In fact, some turn into advocates against diet culture by not participating in diet conversations, challenging mainstream messages (e.g., "slim down for summer"), hosting podcasts, posting anti-diet messages on social media, etc.

There will probably always be pressures related to looks, misguided beliefs about health, and new "fixes" being offered. For example, at the time we are writing this, glucagon-like peptide-1s (GLP-1) for weight loss are quite the rage. They are even being researched as a treatment for some eating disorders.[19] Who knows what will happen—positive or not—in the future? Only time will tell. It can be tricky to discern between something posed as "good for us" versus something that is *actually* good for us. (Remember Fen-phen?) But critical thinking about the miracle drugs, fixes, and potions that society pushes on us is probably one of the strongest protectors of recovery, in our opinion.

Seeing how our clients have been affected by diet culture—also knowing how we were once influenced—has further solidified our critical questioning of marketing and a values shift away from that paradigm. What's more, we know many people who have healed and then chosen to become therapists, dietitians, recovery coaches, peer mentors, etc. Their work has made them even stronger proponents of anti-diet culture. There is hope!

What can I do about social media?

Research has shown body dissatisfaction to be a significant risk factor for those who may develop an eating disorder, a maintaining factor in those who are already struggling, and a potential predictor of relapse in the future.[20] Though it's complex, there's a definite association between social media use and body dissatisfaction.[21]

To comment on the impact of social media on body image and eating as well as how to manage it, we reached out to a colleague, Charlotte Markey, PhD. She's an expert in body image, a professor of psychology, the chair of the health sciences department at Rutgers University, and an author of a series of books on body image. Her most recent book, *Adultish: The Body Image Book for Life*,[22] delves into social media. Below, Dr. Markey shares how social media can harm body image:

> ### *Promoting Unrealistic Appearance Ideals*
>
> Social media often shows only a narrow, heavily edited version of reality, due to filters, airbrushed images, and unattainable beauty standards. Research consistently shows that viewing these "perfect" images can heighten body dissatisfaction, lower mood, and negatively impact eating behaviors and overall mental health.
>
> ### *Encouraging Social Comparison*
>
> A major reason social media can damage body image is that it invites constant comparison. It's natural to compare ourselves to others, but seeing curated images and glamorous lifestyles online can leave many young people feeling like they don't measure up.
>
> ### *Framing Appearance as a "Project"*
>
> Spending too much time on social media can make it seem like our bodies are endless "projects" that require constant improvement. Ads, influencers, and celebrities flood us with products and plans, many of which promote disordered eating behaviors.

Dr. Markey offers her advice on how adults can help:

> ### *Challenge Appearance Ideals and Values*
>
> Adults can protect young people by encouraging them to question the appearance ideals and broader values they see online. Conversations should focus on appreciating people for qualities like kindness, humor, and compassion—not just looks.

It's important to remind teens that attractive appearances without meaningful traits quickly lose their appeal in real life.

Promote Media Literacy

Because teens get so much of their information from social media platforms, it's vital to teach them to approach online content with skepticism. Encourage them to fact-check what they see, look for credible sources, and understand how algorithms influence the content they are exposed to. When teens engage more with reliable, thoughtful content, algorithms can help push more high-quality information their way.

Foster Embodiment

Embodiment means feeling at home in and connected to one's body, and valuing it for what it can do, rather than just how it looks. Adults can encourage embodiment by emphasizing self-care, body trust, and joyful movement. It's also important to model positive behavior ourselves: celebrating our bodies, enjoying food without guilt, getting enough sleep, and avoiding unhealthy habits.

Encourage Intentional Use

Some research suggests that limiting or even taking breaks from social media can help lessen its harmful effects.[23] Still, advising teens to quit social media entirely isn't always realistic—or necessary. Social media isn't all bad; it can also be a source of community, support, and inspiration.[24]

Social media doesn't have to make us feel awful, but it can if we're not careful. People with eating disorders will probably need to protect themselves from the negative effects of social media, especially during recovery. Notice we said protect themselves from, not eliminate, social media. Research shows that adding varied non-body-focused content can improve body image distress and mood.[25] There are ways to use the new norm to your advantage.

We've worked with parents who try to take away their kids' social media or censor their use in some way. This often does not play out well, particularly when the kid is more tech-savvy than the parent (which is almost always). For instance, the child finds a way around the controls, creates a private account under a pseudonym, or blocks the parent on their real account while having a dummy account that their parent can see. That said, we encourage having open and honest conversations about social media, its benefits, and its challenges—as illustrated above by Dr. Markey.

What can I do if my child refuses treatment?

This is so hard on parents! Some won't allow their minor to refuse. However, if the child is an adult or has the legal right to decline, that can be complicated. We've seen various approaches, some successful and others not. We know parents who have considered or taken extreme measures like conservatorships. (If you are considering that, please speak to the clinical team you have in place; they might also point you to a lawyer.) We wish there was a formula that was foolproof and didn't risk damaging relationships. Our best guidance here is to consult with parents, providers, and those with personal experience of eating disorders to figure out *your* most thoughtful approach.

Having said the above, we brainstormed about this conundrum. We share a few scenarios that have helped some individuals with resistance agree to treatment below.

Doctor's Orders

They heard a doctor say, "You need to be admitted," "You're not medically stable," or "I recommend inpatient."

Attending medical appointments as recommended is not only essential to monitor physical safety, but sometimes this kind of unexpected statement from a doctor packs a powerful punch of reality. It can often shake up that anosognosia (seeming unawareness or denial of seriousness). Imagine believing you're "fine," and the medical professional overseeing your care challenges that belief with medical or psychiatric data.

Incentives

They received rewards for going to treatment.

Yes, we know that sounds like bribery. And if it works, so what? Someday, your child may thank you for it. If you decide to use an incentive, it's generally a good idea to involve them in the agreement part. Therefore, they have a stake in it. And make sure you can uphold your end of the bargain. Picture this: You work your tail off for the bonus the company promised, and then the company says, "Nope. Sorry. We can't do that."

Boundary Setting

Their parents (and team, if present) set and followed through with boundaries.

A straightforward example is "I'm not paying for college if you don't get proper help." And you stick to it! Putting boundary contingencies in writing can help keep the eating disorder from revising history or making empty promises to you.

Family Intervention

They were the focus of an intervention staged by their family or a professional.

The range of how an intervention may happen spans widely. For example, Alli has helped families with loving interventions that are extremely different from those you might have seen on television. Surrounding your loved one with the family's vulnerable worry and fear may help them feel the impact their eating disorder is having on others. By experiencing that tidal wave of love, some may want to alleviate the concern and pain of their family members, thus inspiring them to get the help they need.

Communication Improvement

Their parents worked on communication skills.

Effective communication can often help to chip away at the wall that an eating disorder erects. Emotion-focused family therapy (EFFT) has a formula built specifically for piercing through your loved one's defenses and their potentially unclear thinking due to their eating disorder. (See chapter 2, **I'm told what I *shouldn't* say, *but* what *should* I say?** section.) Adele LaFrance, co-developer of EFFT, provides workshops to teach the skills.[26] Alli values LaFrance's work and has seen it make a difference for many families.

Contractual Agreement

They had a say in creating their goals and contingencies.

Let's say your child tells you, "I can do this (recover) without treatment." We encourage you to get detailed about what they are assuring you they will do. Both of you can put it in writing as a contract or goal sheet pertaining to aspects of life and recovery—food, behavioral, relational, physical activity, etc. Think in terms of SMART goals: *S* for specific, *M* for measurable, *A* for achievable, *R* for relevant, and *T* for time-bound.[27]

If they meet their goals, fantastic! Celebrate! But if they don't (e.g., for X number of weeks), that written tracking may build a case for going to treatment, a higher level of care, etc. This tactic can require strategy, and you will probably benefit from professional guidance to execute the process effectively. Contracts are fairly common in eating disorders treatment, but trust us: To create one that is *not* punitive or coercive, *is* clearly defined, provides realistic terms, *and* your loved one agrees to can be an art. If a professional's guidance is not possible, caregivers and those with personal experience of eating disorders will likely be able to offer helpful insight about what's beneficial, harmful, and anywhere in between when utilizing contracts.

Here's an important point about anything mentioned in this section thus far: Take the time to explain *why* something is happening or will happen, and do your best to get their agreement. Each matters for mitigating potential damages from these types of pressuring approaches. Otherwise, your child can feel like things are happening *to* them involuntarily, without their knowledge or consent. And that leads us to the next point being discussed more and more among professionals: harm reduction.

A harm reduction approach focuses on quality of life, not symptom cessation or abstinence. In harm reduction, the person might stay medically compromised, underweight, malnourished, engaging in eating disorder behaviors, etc., while simultaneously trying to reduce the disorder's negative impacts on their life (e.g., the goal could be staying out of the hospital). At this time, harm reduction for eating disorders is viewed as controversial and continues to be studied in the field.[28] Historically, it has generally been reserved for those with severe and enduring anorexia nervosa, which is anorexia nervosa that appears to be treatment-resistant after multiple tries and "state of the art" treatment.[29] We describe it here so you understand the term; it is not typically a starting point for care and is generally used in specific circumstances.

Bottom line: You have a history with your loved one. What do *you* think might get your loved one to agree to treatment? We believe in doing what it takes (within reason while staying ethical, kind, and lawful) to help your child agree to and engage in healing from the eating disorder.

There is no one right answer. That probably isn't what you want to hear, but no matter how deep someone is in their eating disorder, we believe there is a part of them—even if microscopic right now—that does want to heal and have a life without the eating disorder.

What should I do if my loved one doesn't want to recover?

Your job isn't to *make* your loved one want to recover. Your job is to help keep them alive long enough for *them* to want to recover.

Recognize that it's common for people not to want to recover or change, especially at the beginning. Those feelings can also emerge at different times. Yes, this can be a catch-22 of these disorders. Your loved one may, on occasion, seem in denial about the seriousness of their condition, health status, behaviors, etc. That denial may be conscious or unconscious.[30] You may hear your own thoughts screaming at them in frustration, "How can you not see it?!"

Various times, someone quite ill has told Alli—with utter sincerity—that they didn't want to use up a spot that someone *really* sick needed (as if their illness wasn't bad enough to warrant care). That's just one of many ways that denial, missing insight, or failing to realize the severity of their illness shows up and might be a barrier to healing.

As a clinician in private practice, Alli has found the following to be relatively effective in pushing against the "I'm fine"-type response:

> When appropriate, such as someone critically ill needing a higher level of care, I've directly informed them that in my professional opinion, they are *too sick* for me to treat them at an outpatient level of care. They usually protest and minimize their symptoms, and I ask them why I'd be refusing their money when a business's *job* is to make money. (This is one of the rare times I'll put a spotlight on the business aspects of therapy—to challenge their rationale.)
>
> Occasionally, that logic-based question has created enough dissonance to catch their attention and start to build trust. However, their brains are often not being honest with them. Their refusal of appropriate treatment does not necessarily mean that they don't *want* to recover, they may not believe there's a *real* reason or need to.
>
> Additionally, people with eating disorders can have low self-esteem particularly while sick, and I have to be careful that they don't and won't feel that I'm saying *no* because they lack value or worth. More than one has interpreted that a past provider's referral to a higher level of care meant the provider wanted to "get rid" of them, they were not worth it, not likable, etc. It can feel super challenging to navigate the anosognosia (lack of awareness of the seriousness of their condition) even as a professional. (Parents, I hope that normalizes it a bit for you.)

Many people are ambivalent about recovery at best. Some can't imagine themselves as recovered ever. Maybe the eating disorder has become a significant part of their identity, and they don't know who they would be without it. Others would just like to feel a bit better, less strained, or not as consumed by thoughts and behaviors. Wherever they are at, consider starting there, exploring how you might help move the needle toward healing.

What might make my child more invested in their healing and recovery?

In addition to capable treatment being provided or a person's openness to dive in and change, here are some of the strongest influences that we've witnessed.

For Jenny, as a recovery coach, it's a connection with providers, buy-in, and role modeling:

Connection with Providers

To put it bluntly, treatment team providers your kid likes more than their eating disorder. And not "likes" because they can get away with stuff, but those they *respect.* Ideally, your child has enough rapport with their providers that they would rather do the hard things than disappoint. It's not uncommon for kids, teens, and adults with eating disorders to be people pleasers. Sometimes we (you included) can use that trait to help them recover.

Buy-In

This means they are taking an active and participatory role in their treatment. I am such a proponent of *choice.* Here's what I mean: Remember when your child was a toddler? Did you ever let them choose between two outfits? Because going naked was not an option. (And neither was the fashion statement they would invent without any guidance.) It gave them a sense of agency without overwhelming them.

Choices about recovery are similar. For example, your kid can have an option of cuisine, but skipping a meal or snack isn't one of them. They can also have a choice of provider or treatment center, but opting out of treatment isn't a choice. This helps cut the "I didn't have a say in the matter" argument off at the pass.

I've worked with an adolescent who, within twenty-four hours, went from making a sign that said, "F$ck Jenny!" to FaceTiming their friends saying, "Jenny is my new BFF!" (Hold your applause.) And I've worked with others who had similar attitudes before my arrival and then had changes of heart within a short time of working together.

I believe that's because I've been in a position to introduce choice. So often, treatment can feel like it's happening *to* rather than *for* a client. This is particularly true for adolescents, where parents have had to step in as a safety measure.

I ask questions like:

- Is there anything about your relationship to food and exercise that feels less than stellar?
- How can we work together to make it better?
- What do your parents do that feels supportive? And what do they do that doesn't?

In my experience, including them in the process empowers them.

Role Modeling

Most of my clients express tremendous frustration when they are the only one being asked to change. Are there steps you are willing to take in your own personal growth and development that model the kind of work they are being asked to do? If so, please do!

Here's Alli's angle on this as a therapist:

Research consistently shows that the therapeutic alliance is a key factor in successful therapy.[31] It's the relationship a therapist builds with a client—one that can become a foundation for the client's personal growth. I strive to create a safe, attuned space that offers respect, care, opportunities for healthy attachment with ethical boundaries, and a nonjudgmental presence. I bring my knowledge of eating disorders and my training in various therapeutic modalities to support each client's recovery process.

There is almost always something that can help a person move toward healing. My role is to help them find the courage and willingness to try, and to create a space where they feel both safe and cared for as they do so.

The reasons clients consider change are unique to them: the desire to fully play with a beloved pet, the yearning to have a partner someday, a hope to experience college without the eating disorder getting in the way, the willingness to face an unknown future, or the trust that they'll be OK even if they make a "wrong" choice. I don't judge their reasons as significant *enough* or not. Whatever gets (as Jenny said) their buy-in for scary change, yes, let's go with that! (One parent described my approach as gently cracking the door open with hope and possibility—and then jamming my pointy-toe boot in so it can't close again. From there, we push it open, together.)

Many have shared that the illness feels like something they can depend on. Therefore, I know I need to be deeply dependable in the therapeutic relationship. That means showing up solidly and consistently, whether I'm working with the client, a parent, or the family system. I aim to do what I say I'll do; bring authenticity, humor, and humility; and use my skills and training in human (real) and compassionate ways. That kind of steadiness becomes a building block for trust—and your loved one needs to be able to trust something more than they trust the eating disorder.

While there are no guarantees about the outcome, without trust, how can they take the brave steps we ask them to try?

And when they hit sticking points, I'll sometimes remind clients that if they really don't like life in recovery, the eating disorder will still be there—they can always go back to it. And while that sounds a little irreverent, for some it gives just enough permission to take a chance on healing. (For the record, I've never seen anyone prefer their eating disordered life to their full and recovered life.)

In addition to what we've already shared to help a kid, teen, or adult child get more invested in their own healing, rewards and consequences can be used strategically to enhance your child's investment in their recovery process. Historically, has your child been more responsive to rewards or consequences? Can you leverage that?

Insider's tip: If your child is an adolescent, make sure that any recovery-related rewards and consequences are separate from the consequences for "normal" teenage antics and rebellion. Let's say that your child is earning phone privileges through meeting with providers, meal plan completion, etc., and they stay out past their curfew. If you take their phone away for breaking curfew, it's confusing and you lose some leverage! The phone privilege was tied to choosing recovery. What then helps motivate them to participate in treatment?

What if my child has made little to no progress for years?

At this point, you might want to take inventory of all that's been tried so far. Here's an informal assessment that Alli created:

A Reexamination

- What do you think has helped, and why?
- What do you think has not helped, and why?
- What does your loved one think has helped, and why?
- What does your loved one think has not helped, and why?
- What levels of care, modalities, approaches, adjuncts, and support groups have been tried?

- Has there been progress at certain points?
  - Why do you think that was/wasn't happening?
  - Why does your child think that was/wasn't happening?
  - If there are providers included, why do they think that was/wasn't happening?
- Looking back, do you see any patterns? (Those can inform what might need changing.)
- Has your loved one felt included in setting treatment goals and planning?
- Where are they in their willingness to change or heal—meaning, what level of recovery do they want for themselves at this time (e.g., no change at all, a little more freedom from the eating disorder, full recovery, etc.)?

If you don't know what to do or what's possible next, the above questions might help you to figure that out. After this kind of reexamination, Alli has seen parents gain more clarity and revise their plans. For instance, they commit to doing things differently, seeing if there might be positive progress from a changed approach. Or, they decide to repeat something they realized showed progress in the past but maybe wasn't tried long enough.

Talking with your loved one about their experiences and the future they want can provide valuable information. So can brainstorming with people who understand eating disorders (e.g., professionals and support group members) about possible paths forward. (See chapter 1, **How do I find a support group?** section.)

At this point in your journey, you also might feel worn out and want a break. If that's the case, adjust your life as needed for *you* to keep going. That may mean spending time with your other children (if you have them) who have probably not gotten as much attention while the eating disorder has been so hot in the house. Maybe that means reinvesting in hobbies you've had to ignore but could help fill your cup. Perhaps you've missed quality time with a partner or friends.

If you need to step back to recharge, that's human. These disorders can stretch people so very far, and caregiver fatigue is a real thing. Hope can still live inside you—even if you take some distance and rest up after the marathon or sprint you've been doing because you love someone with an eating disorder.

7

Hope and Help

Healing requires humility, curiosity, and openness. Thank you for your time and heart. We close this book with sentiments and tips from others who have been there and us.[1]

What gives Alli and Jenny hope?

So much! But in a nutshell:

From Alli

Regarding people with eating disorders, in my experience, these disorders typically affect powerful human beings, even if they don't yet recognize or are avoiding that strength. I've often found myself wondering if the eating disorder keeps them from stepping into their gifts before they are ready to—*in a strangely protective way.* And that repeated reflection maintains my ongoing hope for them.

Regarding parents and caregivers, what gives me hope is people like you—those who have chosen to walk with their loved one, seeking to understand, assist, and offer compassion when initial impulses could otherwise have driven you apart. It is brave to put yourself in the path of this disorder—to move toward the problem and to grow, even if you didn't necessarily want to. To me, that's inspirational.

Throughout the years, you parents and caregivers have shown me how courageous, persistent, and love-filled you are—that you can often affect positive change even a professional may not be able to create. That fills me with hope and gratitude.

From Jenny

As my recovery coaching clients integrate back into their lives, I'm filled with so much hope. It's an honor to witness them participating in life-affirming activities for the first time without their eating disorders, such as getting a job, going back to school, living independently, dating, and more. It's been especially gratifying when clients return to their passions, such as dance, sports, gymnastics, acting, jewelry making, visual arts, etc.

A while ago, I attended a former client's high school dance performance. When we first started working together post-residential, she avoided a return to dance, despite it being something that she loves. Through the course of our work, she was able to recognize that she was afraid of what it would be like to dance in a weight-restored body. This was something I could deeply empathize with, having gone through similar experiences in my own recovery. Under the guidance of the clinical team, she addressed this fear gradually through exposures—slow, steady, positive reintroductions to movement. I supported her through the process, and she eventually worked up to resuming group classes with her peers.

Seeing her perform for the first time in her recovery was emotional; tear-jerking, to say the least. She expressed so much appreciation for having me there. Lots of hugs were shared. Even though time had passed since working together, there is such a strong connection between us—having both lost and then found a mutual passion, dance.

She made it to the other side, like so many of my clients, and I believe that your kiddo (of any age) can, too!

What do caregivers wish other caregivers knew?

The following messages come to you directly from the parents, spouses, and family members in Alli's caregiver support group. Some messages were originally created for a FEAST blog:[2]

- "You're not alone. You're not the only one experiencing this."
- "All those questions: 'Why didn't I know sooner?' 'Why couldn't I be helpful?' 'What did I do wrong?' It's not your fault."
- "You've got to plug into a network of help because you don't know what you don't know."
- "It's so isolating: the stigma and feeling the need to protect and respect your loved one's privacy. You start with, 'I can't let anyone know in my circles.' Or friends and family you tell don't understand. Find a safe place to connect and share, like a support group, where you can be completely open."
- "When you initially find a group, you're probably in that first-time emotion and uncertainty. From fear, tears, and terror to anger and resentment, it's such a roller coaster. You're overloaded. You are allowed not to know. It's OK to be mad. Give yourself permission to feel all those emotions; all are good and valid."

- "Know that through this journey with your loved one, it is very possible that you will be encouraged, by professionals, to do many things to help your loved one that go against any logic or instinct you had in the past. Many times, those with experience will be correct. The rule book has been changed. That being said, if your spidey senses are tingling because something just doesn't seem right, then give yourself permission to be curious, explore that, and consider making a change."
- "My advice would be to not be scared of the 'right' way to address your child—just address it the first time you notice any 'new or concerning' quirks around eating."
- "I wish I would have watched my own eating habits. They, our children, watch us from the time they are little. All the fad diets mess with their minds, especially as their bodies start going through puberty. It meant a lot to my daughter to watch me throw caution to the wind and eat everything she thought I 'didn't' eat."
- "I would want other parents to know what to look for—negative body image, sudden switch in behavior, skipping meals out of the blue, overexercising, shaming themselves when they eat certain foods. I just wish I had even known a few of these things to look out for. I was completely clueless."
- "There are no easy answers or singular paths."
- "If I got a do-over from the beginning of the diagnosis, I would be so much more aware of my daughter's need for understanding and validation, even if I didn't agree with it. And while that may have been beneficial for her and our relationship, that may not be what every child needs. The journeys are so similar and unique at the same time."

What do kids, teens, and adults wish their parents and caregivers knew?

Jenny contacted people she has known and worked with. Here's what they wished their parents had known, said, or done. Not everything below will apply to your experience. The words and thoughts come directly from people with a variety of eating disorders diagnoses, ages, genders, etc.

The Eating Disorder

- "I wish they knew that at the beginning it was barely even their daughter talking. It was almost always the voice in my head (Ed) talking and engaging with them. I really didn't mean the hurtful and harmful things I said or did to them and myself."
- "I wish my parents would have sat me down and told me how my illness was affecting the family—not in a guilting way, but just so I could see that I wasn't just hurting myself."
- "I wish my parents had known how deadly eating disorders can be and taken a firm and loving approach to getting me help."
- "I wish they knew it's not just the 'sick' person who has work to do. Recovery is made so much easier and less lonely when those around us do their work too."
- "I wish they had known it was an actual disorder and not just stubbornness. I wasn't trying to be difficult, and I didn't want to have these issues."
- "I wish they (my dad specifically) had taken it more seriously and researched the issue instead of blaming me."

- "I wish they had known that eating disorders don't all look the same. I wish they had known what ARFID was and how to help me."
- "I wish my parents would have noticed the signs and researched getting me help at a younger age."
- "I wish my parents would have asked me about my emotional health rather than getting frustrated that I was not eating."
- "I wish that they knew that the eating disorder brings out a very dark side of me. I will lie and lie and lie some more, and yet, none of it is personal or intended to hurt the ones I love."

Weight Stigma

- "I wish my mom had told me: your worth as a person does not rely on how much you weigh or how you look."
- "I wish that they had told me that finding happiness is not related to weight: weight is not a final destination. There are things in life that would fulfill you like friendship, love, and being able to explore with freedom what makes you happy."
- "I wish they would understand that healing from an eating disorder means having a healthier relationship with food and body. It does *not* mean weight loss."
- "I wish that they believed that I am unconditionally allowed to eat and enjoy food regardless of my weight."
- "I wish when my eating disorder started my parents (and doctor too lol) had been aware that I was struggling before I was 'underweight' via my behavior and symptoms instead of waiting for my weight to get low enough to take it seriously."
- "I wish my parents realized that they are impacted by diet culture and dangerous norms around body size."

Treatment Process

- "I wish they knew about compulsive movement. Even though I started eating a good amount and wanted to move, I wish that they would have encouraged me not to, so I could rewire my relationship with movement."
- "I wish they had known that a meal plan is a minimum. I wish they had encouraged me to keep eating past my meal plan when I had extreme hunger—it can be a real thing during the refeeding process. I wish they could have helped me to understand it was normal to eat tons."
- "I wish my parents knew that negative reinforcement wasn't going to make me want to comply with my recovery needs."
- "I wish they knew that most, if not all, eating disorder patients will only get better long term if they choose to do so themselves. No amount of treatment or force can pull someone out of an eating disorder (mentally)."
- "I wish they knew that good days or outcomes do not mean I'm 'cured' and that feeling watched and judged does not make me feel supported."

Physical Appearance

- "I wish my parents had been aware of the way they talked about food and their own bodies in front of me."
- "I wish my parents would have known not to comment on my appearance. Even trying to compliment my body was way too much for me."
- "I wish that they hadn't made so many remarks about attractiveness being based on appearances, which seemed so innocent at the time."

We can imagine that some of the above might feel hard to read. Maybe you have said and done some of the very things these past clients named. Please be gentle with yourself. You have an opportunity moving forward to rewrite the narrative, approaching your own child in different ways and creating new stories.

Closing Thoughts

We hope that through reading this book, you were able to get a bit of a sense of what it might be like to work with a treatment team. You may have noticed some distinctions between the clinical scope of a therapist and the supportive nature of a recovery coach. You might have seen (or hopefully felt) how the roles can work together in service of healing.

Regarding our self-disclosure in this book, not all clinicians or recovery coaches are comfortable with, believe in, or are trained in that. Alli recalls being warned against *any* self-disclosure while in training as a therapist. Still, there are different schools of thought about what's appropriate, and a rule of thumb is this: Self-disclosure must be to benefit the client, not the provider.[3] So that is why we shared the details we did with you, our reader. We hope it felt helpful.

We, as providers, have limited time with your loved one each week relative to all the hours you may spend with them outside of treatment. When we *all* can work collaboratively to surround your child with aligned knowledge, care, support, and messaging, we believe your kid, teen, or adult will have a better chance to heal and eventually thrive.

We recognize that no book can give you a universally applicable response to "What should I do?" or address your *exact* situation. That said, if you consider all the answers in this guide, we believe you will find *your* path.

Keep going. Keep learning. Keep growing. As we mentioned in the "Introduction" of *My Child Has an Eating Disorder: An Essential Guide for Parents of Kids, Teens, and Adults*, there's more information, research, and opinions out there. May you find what resonates most with you and your child.

Your loved one is lucky to have you.

Resources for Caregivers

For your convenience, we've provided an at-a-glance recap of those resources highlighted in these pages. Please refer to the endnotes if what you are seeking is not listed here.

Reading by Contributors to This Book

Costin, Carolyn, and Gwen Schubert Grabb, *8 Keys to Recovery from an Eating Disorder: Effective Strategies from Therapeutic Practice and Personal Experience* (W. W. Norton & Company, 2011).

Costin, Carolyn, and Gwen Schubert Grabb, *8 Keys to Recovery from an Eating Disorder: Workbook* (W. W. Norton & Company, 2017).

Friedman, Jenn, *Veganism and Eating Disorder Recovery* (Routledge, 2022).

Gaudiani, Jennifer L., *Sick Enough: A Guide to the Medical Complications of Eating Disorders and Undernutrition* (Routledge, 2025).

Markey, Charlotte, *Adultish: The Body Image Book for Life* (Cambridge University Press, 2024).

Markey, Charlotte, *Being You: The Body Image Book for Boys* (Cambridge University Press, 2022).

Markey, Charlotte, *The Body Image Book for Girls: Love Yourself and Grow Up Fearless, 2nd ed.* (Cambridge University Press, 2026).

Muhlheim, Lauren, *When Your Teen Has an Eating Disorder: Practical Strategies to Help Your Teen Recover from Anorexia, Bulimia, and Binge Eating* (New Harbinger Publications, 2018).

Muhlheim, Lauren, Jennifer Averyt, and Shannon Patterson, *The Weight-Inclusive CBT Workbook for Eating Disorders: Tools to Reject Diet Culture, Heal Body Shame, and Promote Recovery* (New Harbinger Publications, 2026).

Resch, Elyse, *The Intuitive Eating Journal: Your Guided Journey for Nourishing a Healthy Relationship with Food* (New Harbinger Publications, 2021).

Resch, Elyse, *The Intuitive Eating Workbook for Teens: A Non-Diet, Body Positive Approach to Building a Healthy Relationship with Food* (Instant Help, 2019).

Resch, Elyse, and Evelyn Tribole, *The Intuitive Eating Card Deck: 50 Bite-Sized Ways to Make Peace with Food* (New Harbinger Publications, 2021).

Spotts-De Lazzer, Alli, *MeaningFULL: 23 Life-Changing Stories of Conquering Dieting, Weight, and Body Image Issues* (Unsolicited Press, 2021).

Tribole, Evelyn, and Elyse Resch, *Intuitive Eating*, 4th ed. (St. Martin's Essentials, 2020).

Tribole, Evelyn, and Elyse Resch, *The Intuitive Eating Workbook: Ten Principles for Nourishing a Healthy Relationship with Food*, 2nd ed. (New Harbinger Publications, 2025).

Further Reading

Bulik, Cynthia M., *Midlife Eating Disorders: Your Journey to Recovery* (Walker Books, 2013).

Crosbie, Casey, and Wendy Sterling, *How to Nourish Your Child Through an Eating Disorder: A Simple, Plate-by-Plate Approach® to Rebuilding a Healthy Relationship with Food* (The Experiment, 2018).

Harrison, Christy, *Anti-Diet: Reclaim Your Time, Money, Well-Being, and Happiness Through Intuitive Eating* (Little, Brown Spark, 2019).

Lock, James, and Daniel Le Grange, *Help Your Teenager Beat an Eating Disorder*, 3rd ed. (The Guilford Press, 2025).

Sole-Smith, Virginia, *Fat Talk: Parenting in the Age of Diet Culture* (Henry Holt and Co., 2023).

Thomas, Jennifer J., Kendra R. Becker, and Kamryn T. Eddy, *The Picky Eater's Recovery Book: Overcoming Avoidant/Restrictive Food Intake Disorder* (Cambridge University Press, 2021).

Support Groups and Community

Around the Dinner Table Forum:
https://feast-ed.org/forum/
The Eating Disorder Foundation:
https://eatingdisorderfoundation.org/get-help/support-groups/
Families Empowered and Supporting Treatment of Eating Disorders:
https://feast-ed.org/caregiver-sibling-support-groups

International Eating Disorder Family Support:
https://facebook.com/groups/International.Eating.Disorder.Family.Support.IEDFS
Men of Families Empowered and Supporting Treatment of Eating Disorders:
https://feast-ed.org/men-of-feast
Multi-Service Eating Disorders Association:
https://medainc.org/get-help/free-support-services-drop-in-groups
National Alliance for Eating Disorders:
https://allianceforeatingdisorders.com/groups
National Association for Anorexia Nervosa and Associated Disorders:
https://anad.org/caregiver-or-sibling-support-group-registration-form

Eating Disorders Resource Hubs

Academy for Eating Disorders Publications:
https://aedweb.org/resources/publications
Eating Disorders Information Gateway:
https://allianceforeatingdisorders.com/eating-disorders-gateway
Multi-Service Eating Disorders Association Resources:
https://medainc.org/resources
National Alliance for Eating Disorders Resource Library:
http://allianceforeatingdisorders.com/resource-library
National Eating Disorders Association Grace Holland Cozine Resource Center:
https://nationaleatingdisorders.org/grace-holland-cozine-resource-center-loved-one

Organizations Providing Eating Disorders Information

Academy for Eating Disorders:
https://aedweb.org
Families Empowered and Supporting Treatment of Eating Disorders:
https://feast-ed.org
Multi-Service Eating Disorders Association:
https://medainc.org
National Alliance for Eating Disorders:
https://allianceforeatingdisorders.com

National Association for Anorexia Nervosa and Associated Disorders:
https://anad.org
National Center of Excellence for Eating Disorders:
https://nceedus.org
National Eating Disorders Association:
https://nationaleatingdisorders.org
Project HEAL:
https://theprojectheal.org

Low and No-Fee Support for Your Loved One

Carolyn Costin Institute Coaching Interns:
https://carolyn-costin.com/interns-and-coaches
Centre for Clinical Interventions:
https://cci.health.wa.gov.au
Eating Disorders Anonymous:
https://eatingdisordersanonymous.org
National Alliance for Eating Disorders Helpline:
https://allianceforeatingdisorders.com/find-treatment
National Association for Anorexia Nervosa and Associated Disorders Get Help:
https://anad.org/get-help
National Association for Anorexia Nervosa and Associated Disorders Recovery Mentors:
https://anad.org/get-help/request-a-recovery-mentor
Project HEAL Apply for Treatment Access:
https://theprojectheal.org/apply-for-treatment-access

Insurance Navigation

Centers for Medicare & Medicaid Services Health Insurance Basics:
https://cms.gov/files/document/nsa-health-insurance-basics.pdf
Project HEAL Insurance Navigation Guides:
https://theprojectheal.org/insurance-navigation-guides
Project HEAL Insurance Resource Hub:
https://theprojectheal.org/insurance-resource-hub

Communication Skills

Codependents Anonymous:
https://coda.org
Emotion-Focused Family Therapy (Mental Health Foundations):
https://mentalhealthfoundations.ca
Nonviolent Communication:
https://cnvc.org

Conferences and Events

FEAST of Knowledge:
https://feast-ed.org
International Conference on Eating Disorders:
https://aedweb.org/aed-events
Southern Smash and SmashTALK:
https://allianceforeatingdisorders.com/southern-smash

Notes

Introduction

1 Jon Arcelus, Alex J. Mitchell, and Jackie Wales, "Mortality Rates in Patients With Anorexia Nervosa and Other Eating Disorders: A Meta-Analysis of 36 Studies," *Archives of General Psychiatry* 68, no. 7 (2011): 724–31, https://doi.org/10.1001/archgenpsychiatry.2011.74; Ashlea Hambleton, Genevieve Pepin, Anvi Le, Danielle Maloney, National Eating Disorder Research Consortium, Stephen Touyz et al., "Psychiatric and Medical Comorbidities of Eating Disorders: Findings from a Rapid Review of the Literature," *Journal of Eating Disorders* 10, no. 1 (2022): 132, https://doi.org/10.1186/s40337-022-00654-2; Nadia Micali, "What's Weighing Us Down: Closing the Gap Between the Global Burden of Eating Disorders and Their Representation," *European Child & Adolescent Psychiatry* 31 (2022): 1653–4, https://doi.org/10.1007/s00787-022-02098-0.

2 George Halbeisen, Gerrit Brandt, and Georgios Paslakis, "A Plea for Diversity in Eating Disorders Research," *Frontiers in Psychiatry* 13 (2022): 820043, https://www.frontiersin.org/journals/psychiatry/articles/10.3389/fpsyt.2022.820043.

3 Alli Spotts-De Lazzer and Lauren Muhlheim, "Eating Disorders and Scope of Competence for Outpatient Psychotherapists," *Practice Innovations* 1, no. 2 (2016): 89–104, https://psycnet.apa.org/doi/10.1037/pri0000021; Gabriella Heruc, Kim Hurst, Anjanetta Casey, Kate Fleming, Jeremy Freeman, Anthea Fursland et al., "ANZAED Eating Disorder Treatment Principles and General Clinical Practice and Training Standards," *Journal of Eating Disorders* 8, no. 1 (2020): 63, https://doi.org/10.1186/s40337-020-00341-0.

Chapter 1

1 Amelia Austin, Michaela Flynn, Katie Richards, John Hodsoll, Tiago Antunes Duarte, Paul Robinson, Jonathan Kelly, and Ulrike Schmidt, "Duration of Untreated Eating Disorder and Relationship to Outcomes: A Systematic Review of the Literature," *European Eating Disorders Review* 29, no. 3 (2021): 329–45, https://doi.org/10.1002/erv.2745.

2 Cynthia M. Bulik, *Nine Truths about Eating Disorders* (fact sheet, Academy for Eating Disorders, 2015), https://www.aedweb.org/resources/publications/nine-truths.

3 Katherine Schaumberg, Elisabeth Welch, Lauren Breithaupt, Christopher Hübel, Jessica H. Baker, Melissa A. Munn-Chernoff, Zeynep Yilmaz et al., "The Science Behind the Academy for Eating Disorders' Nine Truths about Eating Disorders," *European Eating Disorders Review* 25, no. 6 (2017): 432–50, https://doi.org/10.1002/erv.2553.

4 Carla Garnett, "The Body Can Rebound: Eating Disorder Damages Are Extensive, But Reversible," *NIH Record* (newsletter) 72, no. 9 (2020), https://nihrecord.nih.gov/2020/05/01/eating-disorder-damages-are-extensive-reversible.

5 *Eating Disorders: What You Need to Know* (National Institute of Mental Health, n.d.), accessed June 10, 2025, https://www.nimh.nih.gov/health/publications/eating-disorders.

6 American Psychiatric Association, "Feeding and Eating Disorders," in *Diagnostic Statistical Manual of Mental Disorders*, 5th ed., text rev. (Washington, DC: American Psychiatric Association, 2022), 381.

7 American Psychiatric Association, "Feeding and Eating Disorders."

8 Alissa A. Haedt-Matt, "Purging Behaviors," in *Encyclopedia of Feeding and Eating Disorders*, ed. Tracey Wade (Singapore: Springer, 2016), https://doi.org/10.1007/978-981-287-087-2_12-1.

9 Anna Keski-Rahkonen and Anu Ruusunen, "Avoidant-Restrictive Food Intake Disorder and Autism: Epidemiology, Etiology, Complications, Treatment, and Outcome," *Current Opinion in Psychiatry* 36, no. 6 (2023): 438–42, https://doi.org/10.1097/YCO.0000000000000896.

10 American Psychiatric Association, "Feeding and Eating Disorders," 376.

11 American Psychiatric Association, "Feeding and Eating Disorders," 392–3.

12 American Psychiatric Association, "Feeding and Eating Disorders," 387–8.

13 American Psychiatric Association, "Feeding and Eating Disorders," 396.

14 American Psychiatric Association, "Feeding and Eating Disorders."

15 American Psychiatric Association, "Feeding and Eating Disorders," 397.

16 Kamryn T. Eddy, David J. Dorer, Debra L. Franko, Kavita Tahilani, Heather Thompson-Brenner, and David B. Herzog, "Diagnostic Crossover in Anorexia Nervosa and Bulimia Nervosa: Implications for DSM-V," *American Journal of Psychiatry* 165, no. 2 (2008): 245–50, https://doi.org/10.1176/appi.ajp.2007.07060951; Riccardo Serra, Chiara Di Nicolantonio, Riccardo Di Febo, Franco De Crescenzo, Johan Vanderlinder, Elske Vrieze et al., "The Transition from Restrictive Anorexia Nervosa to Binging and Purging: A Systematic Review and Meta-Analysis," *Eating and Weight Disorders* 7 (2022): 857–65, https://doi.org/10.1007/s40519-021-01226-0.

17 Müge Arslan, Nurcan Yabancı Ayhan, Esra Tansu Sarıyer, Hatice Çolak, and Ekin Çevik, "The Effect of Bigorexia Nervosa on Eating Attitudes and Physical Activity: A Study on University Students," *International Journal of Clinical Practice* (2022): 6325860, https://doi.org/10.1155/2022/6325860.

18 "Have You Heard About Bigorexia?" National Alliance for Eating Disorders, posted December 30, 2023, https://www.allianceforeatingdisorders.com/have-you-heard-about-bigorexia/.

19 Phillip Aouad, Nerissa Soh, and Stephen Touyz, "Chew and Spit (CHSP): A Systematic Review," *Journal of Eating Disorders* 4 (2016): 23, https://doi.org/10.1186/s40337-016-0115-1.

20 Nina Dittmer, Corinna Jacobi, and Ulrich Voderholzer, "Compulsive Exercise in Eating Disorders: Proposal for a Definition and a Clinical Assessment," *Journal of Eating Disorders* 6 (2018): 42, https://doi.org/10.1186/s40337-018-0219-x.

21 Sohie Elizabeth Coleman and Noreen Caswell, "Diabetes and Eating Disorders: An Exploration of 'Diabulimia,'" *BMC Psychology* 8 (2020): 101, https://doi.org/10.1186/s40359-020-00468-4.

22 Mehmet Fatih Kınık, Ferda Volkan Gönüllü, Zeynep Vatansever, and Işık Karakaya, "Diabulimia, a Type I Diabetes Mellitus-Specific Eating Disorder," *Turk Pediatri Arsivi* 52, no. 1 (2017): 46–9, https://doi.org/10.5152/TurkPediatriArs.2017.2366; "What Exactly Is Diabulimia?" National Alliance for Eating Disorders, posted January 21, 2023, https://www.allianceforeatingdisorders.com/what-exactly-is-diabulimia/?; "Diabulimia," Cleveland Clinic, reviewed January 21, 2025, https://my.clevelandclinic.org/health/diseases/22658-diabulimia.

23 Omer Horovitz and Marios Argyrides, "Orthorexia and Orthorexia Nervosa: A Comprehensive Examination of Prevalence, Risk Factors, Diagnosis, and Treatment," *Nutrients* 15, no. 17 (2023): 3851, https://doi.org/10.3390/nu15173851.

24 Anushua Bhattacharya, Marita Cooper, Carrie McAdams, Rebecka Peebles, and C. Alix Timko, "Cultural Shifts in the Symptoms of Anorexia Nervosa: The Case of Orthorexia Nervosa," *Appetite* 170 (2022): 105869, https://doi.org/10.1016/j.appet.2021.105869.

25 You can find the ICD 10 at https://icd10data.com and the ICD 11 at https://icd.who.int/en. "International Statistical Classification of Diseases and Related Health Problems," 11th ed., World Health Organization, https://icd.who.int/.

26 You can find the DSM at https://appi.org/DSM.

27 *Eating Disorders: A Guide to Medical Care*, 4th ed. (Academy for Eating Disorders, 2021), https://www.aedweb.org/resources/publications/medical-care-standards.

28 Leslie Kaplan, personal communication, n.d.

29 Jennifer L. Gaudiani, *Sick Enough: A Guide to the Medical Complications of Eating Disorders and Undernutrition* (Routledge, 2025). You can find more information about this book at https://www.sickenough.com/.

30 Fauzia Mahr, Pantea Farahmand, Edward O. Bixler, Ronald E. Domen, Eileen M. Moser, Tania Nadeem, Rachel L. Levine, and Katherine A. Halmi, "A National Survey of Eating Disorder Training," *International Journal of Eating Disorders* 48, no. 4 (2015): 443–5, https://doi.org/10.1002/eat.22335.

31 Stacy A. Trent, Maria E. Moreira, Christopher B. Colwell, and Phillip S. Mehler, "ED Management of Patients with Eating Disorders," *American Journal of Emergency Medicine* 31, no. 5 (2013): 859–65, https://doi.org/10.1016/j.ajem.2013.02.035; Connie Ma, Diana Gonzales-Pacheco, Jean Cerami, and Kathryn E. Coakley, "Emergency Medicine Physicians' Knowledge and Perceptions of Training, Education, and Resources in Eating Disorders," *Journal of Eating Disorders* 9 (2021): 4, https://doi.org/10.1186/s40337-020-00355-8.

32 Rachel Goldstein, personal communication, September 19, 2024.

33 You can find EDF support groups at https://eatingdisorderfoundation.org.

34 You can find FEAST support groups at https://feast-ed.org.

35 You can find IEDFS support groups at https://facebook.com/groups/International.Eating.Disorder.Family.Support.IEDFS.

36 You can find MEDA support groups at https://medainc.org.

37 You can find The Alliance support groups at https://allianceforeatingdisorders.com.

38 You can find ANAD support groups at https://anad.org.

39 Sarah Barakat, Siân A. McLean, Emma Bryant, Anvi Le, Peta Marks, National Eating Disorder Research Consortium et al., "Risk Factors for Eating Disorders: Findings from a Rapid Review," *Journal of Eating Disorders* 11 (2023): 8, https://doi.org/10.1186/s40337-022-00717-4.

40 Anna M. Bardone-Cone, Megan B. Harney, Christine R. Maldonado, Melissa A. Lawson, D. Paul Robinson, Roma Smith et al., "Defining Recovery from an Eating Disorder: Conceptualization, Validation, and Examination of Psychosocial Functioning and Psychiatric Comorbidity," *Behaviour Research and Therapy* 43, no. 3 (2010): 194–202, https://doi.org/10.1016/j.brat.2009.11.001.

41 Therese E. Kenny, Kathryn Trottier, and Stephen P. Lewis, "Lived Experience Perspectives on a Definition of Eating Disorder Recovery in a Sample of Predominantly White Women: A Mixed Method Study," *Journal of Eating Disorders* 10 (2022): 149, https://doi.org/10.1186/s40337-022-00670-2.

42 Bardone-Cone et al., "Defining Recovery."

43 Kenny et al., "Lived Experience Perspectives."

44 Carolyn Costin and Gwen Schubert Grabb, *8 Keys to Recovery from an Eating Disorder: Effective Strategies from Therapeutic Practice and Personal Experience* (W. W. Norton & Company, 2011), pp. 16–17.

45 Jane Miskovic-Wheatley, Emma Bryant, Shu Hwa Ong, Sabina Vatter, Anvi Le, National Eating Disorder Research Consortium et al., "Eating Disorder Outcomes: Findings from a Rapid Review of over a Decade of Research" [abstract], *Journal of Eating Disorders* 11 (2023): para. 3, https://doi.org/10.1186/s40337-023-00801-3.

46 Pamela K. Keel, David B. Herzog, Kamryn T. Eddy, Jennifer J. Thomas, Aparna Keshaviah, Nassim Tabri, Helen B. Murray, Elizabeth Hastings, Katherine Edkins, Meera Krishna, and Debra L. Franko, "Recovery from Anorexia Nervosa and Bulimia Nervosa at 22-Year Follow-Up," *Journal of Clinical Psychiatry* 78, no. 2 (2017): 184–9, https://doi.org/10.4088/JCP.15m10393.

Chapter 2

1 "About AED," Academy for Eating Disorders, accessed June 11, 2025, https://www.aedweb.org/about-aed/who-we-are.

2 You can find the information AED offers at https://www.aedweb.org/home.

3 "Who We Are," F.E.A.S.T., accessed June 11, 2025, https://feast-ed.org/our-mission/.

4 You can find the information FEAST offers at https://feast-ed.org/.

5 "Mission & Story," Multi-Service Eating Disorders Association, accessed June 11, 2025, https://medainc.org/about-us/mission-story.

6 You can find the information MEDA offers at https://medainc.org.

7 "About," National Alliance for Eating Disorders, accessed June 11, 2025, https://allianceforeatingdisorders.com/about.

8 You can find the information The Alliance offers at https://allianceforeatingdisorders.com.

9 "Our Mission," National Center of Excellence for Eating Disorders, The University of North Carolina at Chapel Hill, accessed June 11, 2025, https://nceedus.org/about/.

10 You can find the information NCEED offers at https://nceedus.org/.

11 "Our Work," National Eating Disorders Association, accessed June 11, 2025, https://nationaleatingdisorders.org/our-work.

12 You can find the information NEDA offers at https://nationaleatingdisorders.org.

13 "Our Mission," Project HEAL, accessed June 11, 2025, https://www.theprojectheal.org/our-mission.

14 You can find the information PH offers at https://theprojectheal.org.

15 Carolyn Costin and Gwen Schubert Grabb, *8 Keys to Recovery from an Eating Disorder: Effective Strategies from Therapeutic Practice and Personal Experience* (W. W. Norton & Company, 2011). You can find more information about the idea of the eating disorder and healthy self-interplay in the chapter entitled "KEY 2: Your Healthy Self Will Heal Your Eating Disorder Self" (pp. 37–62).

16 Sarah Barakat, Siân A. McLean, Emma Bryant, Anvi Le, Peta Marks, National Eating Disorder Research Consortium et al., "Risk Factors for Eating Disorders: Findings from a Rapid Review," *Journal of Eating Disorders* 11 (2023): 8, https://doi.org/10.1186/s40337-022-00717-4.

17 Selma Øverland Lie, Øyvind Rø, and Lasse Bang, "Is Bullying and Teasing Associated with Eating Disorders? A Systematic Review and Meta-Analysis," *International Journal of Eating Disorders* 52, no. 5 (2019): 497–514, https://doi.org/10.1002/eat.23035; Priscilla dos Reis Oliveira, Marta Angélica Iossi Silva, Wanderle Abadio de Oliveira, André Vilela Komatsu, Marisa Afonso de Andrade Brunherotti, Rafaela Rosário et al., "Associations Between Bullying and Risk for Eating Disorders in Adolescents," *Revista brasileira de enfermagem* 76, no. 5 (2023): e20220643, https://doi.org/10.1590/0034-7167-2022-0643.

18 Dori Rakusin, Kate O'Brien, and Michael Murphy, "Case Reports of New-Onset Eating Disorders in Older Adult Cancer Survivors," *Journal of Eating Disorders* 9 (2021): 166, https://doi.org/10.1186/s40337-021-00522-5.

19 Agnieszka Pelc, Monika Winiarska, Ewelina Polak-Szczybyło, Justyna Godula, and Agnieszka Ewa Stępień, "Low Self-Esteem and Life Satisfaction as a Significant Risk Factor for Eating Disorders Among Adolescents," *Nutrients* 15, no. 7 (2023): 1603, https://doi.org/10.3390/nu15071603.

20 Cara Bohon, Eric Stice, and Emily Burton, "Maintenance Factors for Persistence of Bulimic Pathology: A Prospective Natural History Study," *International Journal of Eating Disorders* 42, no. 2 (2009): 173–8, https://doi.org/10.1002/eat.20600; Walter Kaye, "Neurobiology of Anorexia and Bulimia Nervosa," *Physiology & Behavior* 94 (2008): 121–35, https://doi.org/10.1016/j.physbeh.2007.11.037; Christopher Fairburn, Eric Stice, Zafra Cooper, Helen A. Doll, Patricia A. Norma, and Marianne E. O'Connor, "Understanding Persistence in Bulimia Nervosa: A 5-Year Naturalistic Study," *Journal of Consulting and Clinical Psychology* 71, no. 1 (2003): 103–9, https://psycnet.apa.org/doi/10.1037/0022-006X.71.1.103; Joanna E. Steinglass and B. Timothy Walsh, "Neurobiological Model of the Persistence of Anorexia Nervosa," *Journal of Eating Disorders* 4 (2016): 19, https://doi.org/10.1186/s40337-016-0106-2; Rachel Potterton, Amelia Austin, Karina Allen, Vanessa Lawrence, and Ulrike Schmidt, "'I'm Not a Teenager, I'm 22. Why Can't I Snap Out of It?': A Qualitative Exploration of Seeking Help for a First-Episode Eating Disorder During Emerging Adulthood," *Journal of Eating Disorders* 8 (2020): 46, https://doi.org/10.1186/s40337-020-00320-5.

21 Joseph C. Franklin, Burtrum C. Schiele, Josef Brozek, and Ancel Keys, "Observations on Human Behavior in Experimental Semistarvation and Rehabilitation," *Journal of Clinical Psychology* 4, no. 1 (1948), https://doi.org/10.1002/1097-4679(194801)4:1%3C28::AID-JCLP2270040103%3E3.0.CO;2-F.

22 Cynthia M. Bulik, "Negative Energy Balance: A Biological Trap for People Prone to Anorexia Nervosa," *Exchanges* (blog), UNC Center of Excellence for Eating Disorders, https://uncexchanges.org/2014/12/01/negative-energy-balance-a-biological-trap-for-people-prone-to-anorexia-nervosa/; Kaye, "Neurobiology of Anorexia and Bulimia Nervosa."

23 Sahib S. Khalsa, "Interoception in Eating Disorders: A Clinical Primer," *Psychiatric Times* 36, no. 9 (2019): para. 1, https://www.psychiatrictimes.com/view/interoception-eating-disorders-clinical-primer.

24 E. Martin, C. T. Dourish, P. Rotshtein, M. S. Spetter, and S. Higgs, "Interoception and Disordered Eating: A Systematic Review," *Neuroscience & Biobehavioral Reviews* 109 (2019): 166–91, https://doi.org/10.1016/j.neubiorev.2019.08.020; Carrie Arnold, "A Broken Sense of Self Underlies Eating Disorders," *Scientific American*, published May 1, 2012, https://www.scientificamerican.com/article/inside-the-wrong-body/.

25 Katherine E. Gnall, "Changes in Interoception in Mind-body Therapies for Chronic Pain: A Systematic Review and Meta-Analysis," *International Journal of Behavioral Medicine* 31 (2024): 833–47, https://doi.org/10.1007/s12529-023-10249-z .

26 Yang Yu, Renee Miller, and Susan W. Groth, "A Literature Review of Dopamine in Binge Eating," *Journal of Eating Disorders* 10 (2022): 11, https://doi.org/10.1186/s40337-022-00531-y.

27 Guido K. W. Frank, "The Neurobiology of Eating Disorders," *Child and Adolescent Psychiatric Clinics of North America* 28, no. 4 (2019): 329–40, https://doi.org/10.1016/j.chc.2019.05.007; Guido K. W. Frank, Megan E. Shott, and Joel Stoddard, "Association of Brain Reward Response With Body Mass Index and Ventral Striatal-Hypothalamic Circuitry Among Young Women With Eating Disorders," *JAMA Psychiatry* 78, no. 10 (2021): 1123–33, https://doi.org/10.1001/jamapsychiatry.2021.1580.

28 Claire E. Cusack, "'I'm Still Not Sure If the Eating Disorder Is a Result of Gender Dysphoria': Trans and Nonbinary Individuals' Descriptions of Their Eating and Body Concerns in Relation to Their Gender," *Psychology of*

Sexual Orientation and Gender Diversity 9, no. 4 (2022): 422–33, https://doi.org/10.1037/sgd0000515.

29 Jess Hudgens, personal communication, November 2, 2024.

30 Rachel Bachner-Melman, Yonatan Watermann, Lilac Lev-Ari, and Ada H. Zohar, "Associations of Self-Repression with Disordered Eating and Symptoms of Other Psychopathologies for Men and Women," *Journal of Eating Disorders* 10 (2022): 41, https://doi.org/10.1186/s40337-022-00569-y.

31 You can find more information about CoDA at https://coda.org.

32 "Emotion-Focused Family Therapy," Adele LaFrance, accessed June 11, 2025, https://dradelelafrance.com/efft. You can find more information about EFFT at https://dradelelafrance.com and the sister site https://mentalhealthfoundations.ca.

33 "Resources for Parents and Caregivers," Mental Health Foundations, accessed August 11, 2025, https://mentalhealthfoundations.ca. You can find the instructional videos at https://mentalhealthfoundations.ca/caregivers.

34 "Introduction to NVC," The Center for Nonviolent Communication, accessed June 11, 2025, https://cnvc.org/learn/what-is-nvc. You can find more information about NVC at https://nvc.org.

35 Costin and Grabb, *8 Keys to Recovery*. You can find more information about the concept of traits as assets or liabilities in the chapter titled "Key 3: It's Not About The Food" (pp. 76–82).

36 Trademarks are the property of their respective owner, LucasFilm Ltd.

Chapter 3

1 Deborah Mitchison and Jonathan Mond, "Epidemiology of Eating Disorders, Eating Disordered Behavior, and Body Image Disturbance in Males: A Narrative Review," *Journal of Eating Disorders* 3 (2015): 20, https://doi.org/10.1186/s40337-015-0058-y; Phillipa Hay, Federico Girosi, and Jonathan Mond, "Prevalence and Sociodemographic Correlates of DSM-5 Eating Disorders in the Australian Population," *Journal of Eating Disorders* 3 (2015): 19, https://doi.org/10.1186/s40337-015-0056-0; "Eating Disorders and Males," National Eating Disorders Collaboration, accessed July 9, 2025, https://nedc.com.au/eating-disorders/eating-disorders-explained/eating-disorders-in-males.

2 Jason M. Nagata, Anita V. Chaphekar, Patrick Low, Ruben Vargas, Kyle T. Ganson, Anthony Nguyen et al., "Clinical Characteristics of Hospitalized Male Adolescents and Young Adults with Avoidant/Restrictive Food Intake Disorder (ARFID)." *Journal of Eating Disorders* 13 (2025): 3, https://doi.org/10.1186/s40337-024-01171-0.

3 Sasha Gorrell and Stuart B. Murray, "Eating Disorders in Males," *Child and Adolescent Psychiatric Clinics of North America* 28, no. 4 (2019): 641–51, https://doi.org/10.1016/j.chc.2019.05.012.

4 Sara Bocci Benucci, Giulia Fioravanti, Valeria Silvestro, Maria Chiara Spinelli, Giulietta Brogioni, Aleesia Casalini et al., "The Impact of Following Instagram Influencers on Women's Body Dissatisfaction and Eating Disorder Symptoms," *Nutrients* 16, no. 16 (2024): 2730, https://doi.org/10.3390/nu16162730.

5 Sofie M. Rasmussen, Martin K. Dalgaard, Mia Roloff, Mette Pinholt, Conni Skrubbeltrang, Loa Clausen et al., "Eating Disorder Symptomatology Among Transgender Individuals: A Systematic Review and Meta-Analysis," *Journal of Eating Disorders* 11 (2023): 84, https://doi.org/10.1186/s40337-023-00806-y.

6 Mitchison and Mond, "Epidemiology of Eating Disorders."

7 "Statistics: Eating Disorders," National Institute of Mental Health, accessed June 11, 2025, https://www.nimh.nih.gov/health/statistics/eating-disorders; James I. Hudson, Eva Hiripi, Harrison G. Pope, Jr., and Ronald C. Kessler, "The Prevalence and Correlates of Eating Disorders in the National Comorbidity Survey Replication," *Biological Psychiatry* 61, no. 3 (2006): 348–58, https://doi.org/10.1016/j.biopsych.2006.03.040.

8 Karen L. Samuels, Margo M. Maine, and Mary Tantillo, "Disordered Eating, Eating Disorders, and Body Image in Midlife and Older Women," *Current Psychiatry Reports* 21 (2019): 70, https://doi.org/10.1007/s11920-019-1057-5.

9 Shiri Sadeh-Sharvit, Madeline R. Sacks, Cristin D. Runfola, Cynthia M. Bulik, and James D. Lock, "Interventions to Empower Adults with Eating Disorders and Their Partners Around the Transition to Parenthood," *Family Process* 59, no. 4 (2020): 107–22, https://doi.org/10.1111/famp.12510; Carlos M. Grilo, Maria E. Pagano, Robert L. Stout, John C. Markowitz, Emily B. Ansell, Anthony Pinto et al., "Stressful Life Events Predict Eating

Disorder Relapse Following Remission: Six-Year Prospective Outcomes," *International Journal of Eating Disorders* 45, no. 2 (2012): 185–92, https://doi.org/10.1002/eat.20909.

10 Jessica H. Baker and Cristin D. Runfola, "Eating Disorders in Midlife Women: A Perimenopausal Eating Disorder?" *Maturitas* 85 (2016): 112–16, https://doi.org/10.1016/j.maturitas.2015.12.017; Jody E. Finch, Ziqian Xu, Susan Girdler, and Jessica H. Baker, "Network Analysis of Eating Disorder Symptoms in Women in Perimenopause and Early Postmenopause," *Menopause* 30, no. 3 (2023): 275–82, https://doi.org/10.1097/GME.0000000000002141; Gemma Sharp, Anne Nileshni Fernando, Susan R. Davis, and Alisha Randhawa, "Developing an Educational Resource for People Experiencing Eating Disorders During the Menopause Transition: A Qualitative Co-Design Study," *Journal of Eating Disorders* 12 (2024): 179, https://doi.org/10.1186/s40337-024-01139-0.

11 Rachel Pray and Suzanne Riskin, "The History and Faults of the Body Mass Index and Where to Look Next: A Literature Review," *Cureus* 15, no. 11 (2023): e48230, https://doi.org/10.7759/cureus.48230.

12 "Overweight Olympians: Guess the BMI of Top Athletes," *NewScientist*, published May 15, 2014, https://www.newscientist.com/gallery/obese-olympians/.

13 Keith Devlin, "Top 10 Reasons Why the BMI Is Bogus," *National Public Radio*, published July 4, 2009, https://www.npr.org/2009/07/04/106268439/top-10-reasons-why-the-bmi-is-bogus.

14 You can find more information about #ShakeIt for Self-Acceptance! at https://shakeitforselfacceptance.com.

15 Aikaterini Palascha, Ellen van Kleef, and Hans CM van Trijp, "How Does Thinking in Black and White Terms Relate to Eating Behavior and Weight Gain?" *Journal of Health Psychology* 20 (2015): 638–48, https://doi.org/10.1177/1359105315573440; Bruno Bonfá-Araujo, Atsushi Oshio, and Nelson Hauck-Filho, "Seeing Things in Black-and-White: A Scoping Review on Dichotomous Thinking Style," *Japanese Psychological Research*, 64 (2022): 461–72, https://doi.org/10.1111/jpr.12328.

16 Andrea E. Hamel, Shannon L. Zaitsoff, Andrew Taylor, Rosanne Menna, and Daniel Le Grange, "Body-Related Social Comparison and Disordered Eating among Adolescent Females with an Eating Disorder, Depressive

Disorder, and Healthy Controls," *Nutrients* 4, no. 9 (2012): 1260–72, https://doi.org/10.3390/nu4091260.

17 Alli Spotts-De Lazzer, *MeaningFULL: 23 Life-Changing Stories of Conquering Dieting, Weight, & Body Image Issues* (Unsolicited Press, 2021). You can find more information at https://www.meaningfullread.com/ and https://www.liveyourfullstory.com/books.

18 Carolyn Costin and Gwen Schubert Grabb, *8 Keys to Recovery from an Eating Disorder Workbook* (W. W. Norton & Company, 2017), 132–5.

19 Minor wording changes to the assessment questions are indicated by brackets. Please note that we modified the instructions and abridged the scoring section.

20 Evelyn Tribole and Elyse Resch, *Intuitive Eating: A Revolutionary Anti-Diet Approach*, 4th ed. (St. Martin's Essentials, 2020).

21 Elyse Resch, personal communication, July 23, 2024.

22 "10 Principles of Intuitive Eating," The Original Intuitive Eating Pros, accessed June 10, 2025, https://intuitiveeating.org/about-us/10-principles-of-intuitive-eating.

23 Tribole and Resch, *Intuitive Eating*; Tribole and Elyse, *The Intuitive Eating Workbook: Ten Principles for Nourishing a Healthy Relationship with Food* (New Harbinger Publications, 2021); Resch, *The Intuitive Eating Workbook for Teens: A Non-Diet, Body Positive Approach to Building a Healthy Relationship with Food* (Instant Help, 2019); Resch, *The Intuitive Eating Journal: Your Guided Journey for Nourishing a Healthy Relationship with Food* (New Harbinger Publications, 2021); Resch and Tribole, *The Intuitive Eating Card Deck: 50 Bite-Sized Ways to Make Peace with Food* (New Harbinger Publications, 2021). You can find additional Intuitive Eating publications at https://intuitiveeating.org/our-books.

24 Casey Crosby and Wendy Sterling, *How to Nourish Your Child Through an Eating Disorder: A Simple Plate-by-Plate Approach to Rebuilding a Healthy Relationship with Food* (The Experiment, 2018). You can find more information on this book and the Plate-by-Plate Approach at https://platebyplateapproach.com.

25 "Rebuilding a Healthy Relationship with Food," Plate-by-Plate Approach, accessed June 10, 2025, https://www.platebyplateapproach.com/.

Chapter 4

1 Michael Lutter, *Gifted: Genetic Information for Treating Eating Disorders* (Michael Lutter, 2023).

2 Timothy D. Brewerton, Kim Dennis, and David A. Wiss, "Dismantling the Myth of 'All Foods Fit' in Eating Disorder Treatment," *Journal of Eating Disorders* 12 (2024): 60, https://doi.org/10.1186/s40337-024-01017-9.

3 Ernest Mas-Herrero, Alain Dagher, Marcel Farrés-Franch, and Robert J. Zatorre, "Unraveling the Temporal Dynamics of Reward Signals in Music-Induced Pleasure with TMS," *Journal of Neuroscience* 41, no. 17, 3889–99, https://doi.org/10.1523/JNEUROSCI.0727-20.2020.

4 For more information, see Paul C. Fletcher and Paul J. Kenny, "Food Addiction: A Valid Concept?" *Neuropsychopharmacology* 43 (2018): 2506–13, https://doi.org/10.1038/s41386-018-0203-9; Ashley N. Gearhardt and Johannes Hebebrand, "The Concept of 'Food Addiction' Helps Inform the Understanding of Overeating and Obesity: Debate Consensus," *The American Journal of Clinical Nutrition* 113, no. 2 (2021): 274–6, https://doi.org/10.1093/ajcn/nqaa345.

5 American Psychiatric Association, *Diagnostic and Statistical Manual of Mental Disorders*, 5th ed., text revision (American Psychiatric Publishing, 2022).

6 Michael Lutter, personal communication, November 29, 2024. Joseph C. Franklin, Burtrum C. Schiele, Josef Brozek, and Ancel Keys, "Observations on Human Behavior in Experimental Semi-Starvation and Rehabilitation," *Journal of Clinical Psychology* 4, no. 1 (1948): 28–45, https://doi.org/10.1002/1097-4679(194801)4:1%3C28::AID-JCLP2270040103%3E3.0.CO;2-F; Margaret L. Westwater, Paul C. Fletcher, and Hisham Ziauddeen, "Sugar Addiction: The State of the Science," *European Journal of Nutrition* 55, suppl. 2 (2016): 55–69, https://doi.org/10.1007/s00394-016-1229-6.

7 Sinead Day, Deborah Mitchison, Haider Mannan, W. Kathy Tannous, Janet Conti, Amanda Dearden et al., "Residential Versus Day Program for Eating Disorders: A Comparison of Post-Treatment Outcomes and Predictors," *Journal of Affective Disorders* 371 (2025): 177–86, https://doi.org/10.1016/j.jad.2024.11.054.

8 "Inpatient vs. Residential Eating Disorder Treatment: How to Determine Which Is Necessary," Eating Disorder Hope, published September 11, 2024,

https://www.eatingdisorderhope.com/treatment-for-eating-disorders/types-of-treatments/inpatient-vs-residential.

9 American Psychiatric Association, *American Psychiatric Association Practice Guideline for the Treatment of Patients with Eating Disorders*, 4th ed. (American Psychiatric Association, 2023), https://psychiatryonline.org/doi/book/10.1176/appi.books.9780890424865.

10 You can find out more about the levels of care by watching "Demystifying Higher Levels of Care for Eating Disorders," posted August 29, 2023, by NCEED NC, YouTube, https://www.youtube.com/watch?v=jzZeoEijaD4.

11 Christopher G. Fairburn, *Cognitive Behavior Therapy and Eating Disorders* (Guilford Press, 2008).

12 American Psychiatric Association, *Practice Guideline for Treatment*; Renee D. Rienecke and Daniel Le Grange, "The Five Tenets of Family-based Treatment for Adolescent Eating Disorders," *Journal of Eating Disorders* 10 (2022): 60, https://doi.org/10.1186/s40337-022-00585-y; Svetlana Oshukova, Jaana Suokas, Mai Nordberg, and Monica Ålgars, "Effects of Family-Based Treatment on Adolescent Outpatients Treated for Anorexia Nervosa in the Eating Disorder Unit of Helsinki University Hospital," *Journal of Eating Disorders* 11 (2023): 154, https://doi.org/10.1186/s40337-023-00879-9.

13 Alexa L'Insalata, Claire Trainor, Cara Bohon, Sangeeta Mondal, Daniel Le Grange, and James Lock, "Confirming the Efficacy of an Adaptive Component to Family-Based Treatment for Adolescent Anorexia Nervosa: Study Protocol for a Randomized Controlled Trial," *Frontiers in Psychiatry* 11 (2020): 41, https://doi.org/10.3389/fpsyt.2020.00041.

14 Peter M. Doyle, Daniel Le Grange, Katharine Loeb, Angela Celio Doyle, and Ross D. Crosby, "Early Response to Family-Based Treatment for Adolescent Anorexia Nervosa," *International Journal of Eating Disorders* 43, no. 7 (2010): 659–62, https://doi.org/10.1002/eat.20764; Jessica L. Van Huysse, Kellsey Smith, Kathleen A. Mammel, Natalie Prohaska, and Renee D. Rienecke, "Early Weight Gain Predicts Treatment Response in Adolescents with Anorexia Nervosa Enrolled in a Family-Based Partial Hospitalization Program," *International Journal of Eating Disorders* 53, no. 4 (2020): 606–10, https://doi.org/10.1002/eat.23248.

15 James Lock and Daniel Le Grange, *Help Your Teenager Beat an Eating Disorder* (The Guilford Press, 2017); Lauren Muhlheim, *When Your Teen*

Has an Eating Disorder: Practical Strategies to Help Your Teen Recover from Anorexia, Bulimia, and Binge Eating (New Harbinger Publications, 2018).

16 Lars-Göran Öst, Martin Brattmyr, Anna Finnes, Ata Ghaderi, Audun Havnen, Maria Hedman-Lagerlöf et al., "Cognitive Behavior Therapy for Adult Eating Disorders in Routine Clinical Care: A Systematic Review and Meta-Analysis," *International Journal of Eating Disorders* 57, no. 2 (2024): 249–64, https://doi.org/10.1002/eat.24104; American Psychiatric Association, *Practice Guideline for Treatment.*

17 American Psychiatric Association, *Practice Guideline for Treatment.*

18 Christopher G. Fairburn et al., "A Transdiagnostic Comparison of Enhanced Cognitive Behaviour Therapy (CBT-E) and Interpersonal Psychotherapy in the Treatment of Eating Disorders," *Behaviour Research and Therapy* 70 (2015): 64–71, https://doi.org/10.1016/j.brat.2015.04.010.

19 Eva Vall and Tracey D. Wade, "Predictors of Treatment Outcome in Individuals with Eating Disorders: A Systematic Review and Meta-Analysis," *International Journal of Eating Disorders* 48, no. 7 (2015): 946–71, https://doi.org/10.1002/eat.22411.

20 Lauren Muhlheim, Jennifer Averyt, and Shannon Patterson, *The Weight-Inclusive CBT Workbook for Eating Disorders: Tools to Reject Diet Culture, Heal Body Shame, and Promote Recovery* (New Harbinger Publications, 2026).

21 Lauren Muhlheim, personal communication, August 4, 2024.

22 S. P. Anusuya and S. Gayatridevi, "Acceptance and Commitment Therapy and Psychological Well-Being: A Narrative Review," *Cureus* 17, no. 1 (2025), https://doi.org/10.7759/cureus.77705.

23 Suma P. Chand, Daniel P. Kuckel, and Martin R. Huecker, "Cognitive Behavior Therapy," StatPearls, National Library of Medicine, updated May 23, 2023, https://www.ncbi.nlm.nih.gov/books/NBK470241/.

24 Jennifer J. Thomas, Elizabeth A. Lawson, Nadia Micali, Madhusmita Misra, Thilo Deckersbach, and Kamryn T. Eddy, "Avoidant/Restrictive Food Intake Disorder: A Three-Dimensional Model of Neurobiology with Implications for Etiology and Treatment," *Current Psychiatry* 19 (2017): 57, https://doi.org/10.1007/s11920-017-0795-5.

25 Julie Corliss, "Dialectical Behavior Therapy: What Is It and Who Can It Help?" Harvard Health Publishing, published January 22, 2024, https://www

.health.harvard.edu/blog/dialectical-behavior-therapy-what-is-it-and-who-can-it-help-202401223009.

26 "What Is EMDR Therapy?" EMDR Institute, Inc., accessed December 3, 2024, https://www.emdr.com/what-is-emdr/.

27 Dianne M. Hezel and H. Blair Simpson, "Exposure and Response Prevention for Obsessive-Compulsive Disorder: A Review and New Directions," *Indian Journal of Psychiatry* 61, suppl. 1 (2019): S85–S92, https://doi.org/10.4103/psychiatry.IndianJPsychiatry_516_18.

28 "Integrative Cognitive Affective Therapy (ICAT)," New Zealand Eating Disorders Clinic, accessed December 3, 2024, https://www.nzeatingdisordersclinic.co.nz/treatments/integrative-cognitive-affective-therapy-icat/.

29 IFS Institute, accessed December 3, 2024, https://www.ifs-institute.com/.

30 "Overview of IPT," ISIPT, accessed December 3, 2024, https://interpersonalpsychotherapy.org/ipt-basics/overview-of-ipt/.

31 Kiayuan Zhang, Qihang Xie, Chuan Fan, Xinyang Hu, Jianxiang Lei, Jiacheng Kong et al., "The Effectiveness of Interpersonal Psychotherapy Versus Cognitive Behavioural Therapy for Eating Disorders: A Systematic Review and Meta-Analysis," *Clinical Psychology & Psychotherapy* 31, no. 1 (2024): e2953, https://doi.org/10.1002/cpp.2953; Catherine Crone, Laura J. Fochtmann, Evelyn Attia, Robert Boland, Javier Escobar, Victor Fornari, Neville Golden et al., "The American Psychiatric Association Practice Guideline for the Treatment of Patients With Eating Disorders," *American Journal of Psychiatry* 180, no. 2 (February 2023): 167–71, https://doi.org/10.1176/appi.ajp.23180001.

32 "Psychodynamic Therapy," Psychology Today, updated April 28, 2022, https://www.psychologytoday.com/us/therapy-types/psychodynamic-therapy.

33 Academy for Eating Disorders, *The AED Guide to Selecting Pharmacologic Treatments for Patients with Eating Disorders* (Academy for Eating Disorders, accessed June 18, 2025), https://www.aedweb.org/resources/publications.

34 Amaani H. Hatoum and Amy L. Burton, "Applications and Efficacy of Radically Open Dialectical Behavior Therapy (RO DBT): A Systematic Review of the Literature," *Journal of Clinical Psychology* 80, no. 11 (2024): 2283–302, https://doi.org/10.1002/jclp.23735.

35 Marie Kuhfuß, Tobias Maldei, Andreas Hetmanek, and Nicola Baumann, "Somatic Experiencing – Effectiveness and Key Factors of a Body-Oriented Trauma Therapy: A Scoping Literature Review," *European Journal of Psychotraumatology* 12, no. 1 (2021): 1929023, https://doi.org/10.1080/20008198.2021.1929023.

36 Sinead Day, Phillipa Hay, Kathy Tannous Wadad, Scott J. Fatt, and Deborah Mitchison, "A Systematic Review of the Effect of PTSD and Trauma on Treatment Outcomes for Eating Disorders," *Trauma, Violence, & Abuse* 25, no. 2 (2024): 947–64, https://doi.org/10.1177/15248380231167399.

37 "Trauma," American Psychological Association, accessed June 18, 2025, https://www.apa.org/topics/trauma.

38 Elyssa Barbash, "Different Types of Trauma: Small 't' versus Large 'T,'" Psychology Today, March 13, 2017, https://www.psychologytoday.com/us/blog/trauma-and-hope/201703/different-types-trauma-small-t-versus-large-t.

39 Bessel van der Kolk, *The Body Keeps the Score: Brain, Mind, and Body in the Healing of Trauma* (Penguin Books, 2015); Resmaa Menakam, *My Grandmother's Hands: Racialized Trauma and the Pathway to Mending Our Hearts and Bodies* (Central Recovery Press, 2017).

40 Stuart B. Murray, Eva Pila, Scott Griffiths, and Daniel Le Grange, "When Illness Severity and Research Dollars Do Not Align: Are We Overlooking Eating Disorders?" *World Psychiatry* 16, no. 3 (2017): 321, https://doi.org/10.1002/wps.20465.

41 Georg Halbeisen, Gerrit Brandt, and Georgios Paslakis, "A Plea for Diversity in Eating Disorders Research," *Frontiers in Psychiatry* 13 (2022): 820043, https://doi.org/10.3389/fpsyt.2022.820043.

42 Susan M. Byrne and Anthea Fursland, "New Understandings Meet Old Treatments: Putting a Contemporary Face on Established Protocols," *Journal of Eating Disorders* 12 (2024): 26, https://doi.org/10.1186/s40337-024-00983-4; Halbeisen et al., "A Plea for Diversity."

43 Thomas Ostermann, Hannah Vogel, Katja Boehm, and Holger Cramer, "Effects of Yoga on Eating Disorders—A Systematic Review," *Complementary Therapies in Medicine* 46 (2019): 73–80, https://doi.org/10.1016/j.ctim.2019.07.021.

44 You can find more information about Eat Breathe Thrive at https://www.eatbreathethrive.org.

45 Chelsea Roff, personal communication, August 6, 2024.

46 Jianan Zhong et al., "The Efficacy of Internet-Based Cognitive Behavioral Therapy for Adult Binge Spectrum Eating Disorders: A Meta-Analysis," *Journal of Affective Disorders* 361 (2024): 684–92, https://doi.org/10.1016/j.jad.2024.06.084; Elnaz Moghimi, Caroline Davis, and Michael Rotondi, "The Efficacy of eHealth Interventions for the Treatment of Adults Diagnosed With Full or Subthreshold Binge Eating Disorder: Systematic Review and Meta-Analysis," *Journal of Medical Internet Research* 23, no. 7 (2021): e17874, https://doi.org/10.2196/17874; Dori Steinberg, Taylor Perry, David Freestone, Cara Bohon, Jessica H. Baker, and Erin Parks, "Effectiveness of Delivering Evidence-Based Eating Disorder Treatment via Telemedicine for Children, Adolescents, and Youth," *Eating Disorders* 31, no. 1 (2023): 85–101, https://doi.org/10.1080/10640266.2022.2076334.

47 Catherine Stewart, Anna Konstantellou, Fatema Kassamali, Natalie McLaughlin, Darren Cutinha, Rachel Bryant-Waugh et al., "Is This the 'New Normal'? A Mixed Method Investigation of Young Person, Parent and Clinician Experience of Online Eating Disorder Treatment During the COVID-19 Pandemic," *Journal of Eating Disorders* 9 (2021): 78, https://doi.org/10.1186/s40337-021-00429-1.

48 Christoph Flükiger, A. C. Del Re, Bruce E. Wampold, and Adam O. Horvath, "The Alliance in Adult Psychotherapy: A Meta-Analytic Synthesis," *Psychotherapy* 55, no. 4 (2018): 316–20, https://doi.org/10.1037/pst0000172.

49 National Eating Disorders Association, "Questions to Ask Treatment Providers," accessed June 18, 2025, https://nationaleatingdisorders.org/questions-to-ask-treatment-providers.

50 WebMD Editorial Contributor, "DO vs. MD: What's the Difference?" reviewed by Jabeen Begum, WebMD, published July 18, 2024, https://www.webmd.com/a-to-z-guides/difference-between-md-and-do.

51 Timothy M. Smith, "What's the Difference Between Physician Assistants and Physicians?" American Medical Association, published December 4, 2023, https://www.ama-assn.org/practice-management/scope-practice/whats-difference-between-physician-assistants-and-physicians.

52 Alli Spotts-De Lazzer and Lauren Muhlheim, "Eating Disorders and Scope of Competence for Outpatient Psychotherapists," *Practice Innovations* 1, no. 2 (2016): 89–104, https://psycnet.apa.org/doi/10.1037/pri0000021.

53 Heather Thompson-Brenner, Dana A. Satir, Debra L. Franko, and David B. Herzog, "Clinician Reactions to Patients With Eating Disorders: A Review of the Literature," *Psychiatric Services* 63 no. 1 (2012): 73–8, https://doi.org/10.1176/appi.ps.201100050.

54 *Health Insurance Basics* (Centers for Medicaid & Medicaid Services, revised September 2023), https://www.cms.gov/files/document/nsa-health-insurance-basics.pdf.

55 Rachel Presskreischer, personal communication, August 4, 2024.

56 You can find Project HEAL's insurance resource hub at https://theprojectheal.org/insurance-resource-hub and insurance navigation guides at https://theprojectheal.org/insurance-navigation-guides.

57 Jennifer L. Gaudiani, *Sick Enough: A Guide to the Medical Complications of Eating Disorders and Undernutrition* (Routledge, 2025).

58 Jennifer Gaudiani, personal communication, August 31, 2024.

Chapter 5

1 American Psychiatric Association, *American Psychiatric Association Practice Guideline for the Treatment of Patients with Eating Disorders*, 4th ed. (American Psychiatric Publishing, 2023).

2 Kristen Weir, "New Insights on Eating Disorders," *Monitor on Psychology* 47, no. 4 (2016): 36, https://www.apa.org/monitor/2016/04/eating-disorders.

3 Vikas Duvvuri, personal communication, September 17, 2024.

4 Eva Musby, "How to Tell the School of Your Child's Eating Disorder Needs: Template for a 504 Plan," Anorexia Family, updated December 9, 2024, at https://anorexiafamily.com/template-504-plan-school-eating-disorder.

5 Danika A. Quesnel, Marita Cooper, Maria Fernandez-del-Valle, Alanah Reilly, and Rachel M. Calogero, "Medical and Physiological Complications of Exercise for Individuals with an Eating Disorder: A Narrative Review," *Journal of Eating Disorders* 11 (2023): 3, https://doi.org/10.1186/s40337-022-00685-9.

6 Brian J. Cook, Stephen A. Wonderlich, James E. Mitchell, Ron Thompson, Roberta Sherman, and Kimberli McCallum, "Exercise in Eating Disorders

Treatment: Systematic Review and Proposal of Guidelines," *Medicine & Science in Sports & Exercise* 48, no. 7 (2016): 1408–14, https://doi.org/10.1249/MSS.0000000000000912.

7 Rachel M. Calogero and Kelly N. Pedrotty, "The Practice and Process of Healthy Exercise: An Investigation of the Treatment of Exercise Abuse in Women with Eating Disorders," *Eating Disorders* 12, no. 4 (2004): 273–91, https://doi.org/10.1080/10640260490521352; Maria Fernandez-del-Valle, Eneko Larumbe-Zabala, Angel Villaseñor-Montarroso, Claudia Cardona Gonzalez, Ingnacio Diez-Vega, Luis Miguel Lopez Mojares et al., "Resistance Training Enhances Muscular Performance in Patients with Anorexia Nervosa: A Randomized Controlled Trial," *International Journal of Eating Disorders* 47, no. 6 (2014): 601–9, https://doi.org/10.1002/eat.22251; Brian J. Cook and Heather A. Hausenblas, "Eating Disorder-Specific Health-Related Quality of Life and Exercise in College Females," *Quality of Life Research* 20 (2011): 1385–90, https://doi.org/10.1007/s11136-011-9879-6; Mori J. Krantz, Jennifer L. Gaudiani, Victor W. Johnson, and Philip S. Mehler, "Exercise Electrocardiography Extinguishes Persistent Junctional Rhythm in a Patient with Severe Anorexia Nervosa," *Cardiology* 120, no. 4 (2012): 217–20, https://doi.org/10.1159/000335481.

8 Quesnel et al., "Medical and Physiological Complications of Exercise for Individuals with an Eating Disorder," 3.

9 Cook et al., "Exercise in Eating Disorders Treatment"; Danika A. Quesnel, Brian Cook, and Cristina Caperchione, "Guiding Principles to Inform Future Exercise Protocols for Eating Disorder Treatment," *Health & Fitness Journal of Canada* 13, no. 2 (2020), https://doi.org/10.14288/hfjc.v13i2.297.

10 Quesnel et al., "Guiding Principles to Inform Future Exercise."

11 Jenn Friedman, *Veganism and Eating Disorder Recovery* (Routledge, 2022).

12 "Definition of Veganism," The Vegan Society, accessed June 18, 2025, https://www.vegansociety.com/go-vegan/definition-veganism.

13 Jenn Friedman, personal communication, May 26, 2025.

14 American Psychiatric Association, *Practice Guideline for Treatment.*

15 J. O. Prochaska and C. C. DiClemente, "Stages and Processes of Self-Change of Smoking: Toward an Integrative Model of Change," *Journal of Consulting and Clinical Psychology* 51, no. 3 (1983): 395, https://psycnet.apa.org/doi/10.1037/0022-006X.51.3.390; Nahrain Raihan and Mark Cogburn, StatPearls,

National Library of Medicine, updated March 6, 2023, https://www.ncbi.nlm.nih.gov/books/NBK556005/.

16 "Stages of Change," National Eating Disorders Collaboration, accessed June 18, 2025, https://nedc.com.au/eating-disorders/treatment-and-recovery/stages-of-change.

Chapter 6

1 You can find a list of CCI coaching interns who are providing no-cost sessions at https://carolyn-costin.com/interns-and-coaches.

2 Eating Disorders Anonymous, https://eatingdisordersanonymous.org/. You can find EDA meetings at https://eatingdisordersanonymous.org/meetings/.

3 You can find lower-fee treatment options through The Alliance at https://allianceforeatingdisorders.com/find-treatment.

4 "Eating Disorder Peer Support Groups," National Association of Anorexia Nervosa and Associate Disorders, accessed June 18, 2025, https://anad.org/get-help/about-our-support-groups/.

5 You can find free support services ANAD offers at https://anad.org/get-help.

6 You can find how to connect with a recovery mentor from ANAD at "Request a Recovery Mentor," https://anad.org/get-help/request-a-recovery-mentor.

7 You can find Treatment Access applications for treatment placement and cash assistance that Project HEAL offers at https://theprojectheal.org/apply-for-treatment-access.

8 Centre for Clinical Interventions, *Break Free from ED*, updated July 13, 2022, https://www.cci.health.wa.gov.au/Resources/For-Clinicians/Eating-Disorders.

9 Emily T. Troscianko, Rocío Riestra-Camacho, and James Carney, "Ethics-Testing an Eating Disorder Recovery Memoir: A Pre-Publication Experiment," *Journal of Eating Disorders* 12 (2024): 114, https://doi.org/10.1186/s40337-024-01060-6.

10 Troscianko et al., "Ethics-Testing an Eating Disorder Recovery Memoir."

11 Lauren Muhlheim and Alli Spotts-De Lazzer, "Having Trouble Finding an Eating Disorder Therapist Who Takes Insurance? Here's Why," Kantor & Kantor, posted December 15, 2016, https://www.kantorlaw.net/having-trouble-finding-an-eating-disorder-therapist-who-takes-insurance-heres-why/.

12 Tracey D. Wade, Roz Shafran, and Zafra Cooper, "Developing a Protocol to Address Co-occurring Mental Health Conditions in the Treatment of Eating Disorders," *International Journal of Eating Disorders* 57, no. 6 (2024): 1291–9, https://onlinelibrary.wiley.com/doi/10.1002/eat.24008.

13 Ashlea Hambleton, Genevieve Pepin, Anvi Le, Danielle Maloney, National Eating Disorder Research Consortium, Stephen Touyz, and Sarah Maquire, "Psychiatric and Medical Comorbidities of Eating Disorders: Findings from a Rapid Review of the Literature," *Journal of Eating Disorders* 10 (2022): 132, https://doi.org/10.1186/s40337-022-00654-2.

14 Manja M. Engel, E. M. Woertman, H. C. Dijkerman, and A. Keizer, "Functionality Appreciation Is Associated with Improvements in Positive and Negative Body Image in Patients with an Eating Disorder and Following Recovery," *Journal of Eating Disorders* 11 (2023): 179, https://doi.org/10.1186/s40337-023-00903-y.

15 "From New York to Instagram: The History of the Body Positivity Movement," BBC, accessed June 18, 2025, https://www.bbc.co.uk/bitesize/articles/z2w7dp3.

16 Nichole L. Wood-Barcalow, Jessica M. Alleva, and Tracy L. Tylka, "Revisiting Positive Body Image to Demonstrate How Body Neutrality Is Not New," *Body Image* 50 (2024): 101741, https://doi.org/10.1016/j.bodyim.2024.101741.

17 Charlotte Markey, *Adultish: The Body Image Book for Life* (Cambridge University Press, 2024).

18 Wood-Barcalow et al., "Revisiting Body Image"; Jake Linardon, Zoe McClure, Tracy L. Tylka, and Matthew Fuller-Tyszkiewicz, "Body Appreciation and Its Psychological Correlates: A Systematic Review and Meta-Analysis," *Body Image* 42 (2022): 287–96, https://doi.org/10.1016/j.bodyim.2022.07.003; Engel et al., "Functionality Appreciation Is Associated with Improvements in Positive and Negative Body Image in Patients with an Eating Disorder and Following Recovery," 179; Leesa M. Van Niekerk, Gemma Muscella, and Michael Quinn, "A Validation of the Body Compassion Scale in Females," *Journal of Health Psychology* 28, no. 10

(2023): 900–12, https://doi.org/10.1177/13591053231160922; Jennifer Paff Ogle, Ashlie N. Johnson, Kelly L. Reddy-Best, Jennifer Harmon, Kristen Morris, and Piper Kitterson, "A Qualitative Exploration of Positive Body Image Experiences Among Nonbinary Individuals," *Body Image* 47 (2023): 101632, https://doi.org/10.1016/j.bodyim.2023.101632; Markey, *Adultish: The Body Image Book.*

19 Sara Bartel, Susan L. McElroy, Danielle Levangie, and Aaron Keshen, "Use of Glucagon-Like Peptide-1 Receptor Agonists in Eating Disorder Populations," *International Journal of Eating Disorders* 57, no. 2 (2024): 286–93, https://doi.org/10.1002/eat.24109.

20 Elizabeth H. Evans, Martin J. Tovée, Lynda G. Boothroyd, and Robert F. Drewett, "Body Dissatisfaction and Disordered Eating Attitudes in 7- to 11-Year-Old Girls: Testing a Sociocultural Model," *Body Image* 10, no. 1 (2013): 8–15, https://doi.org/10.1016/j.bodyim.2012.10.001; Paul Rohde, Eric Stice, and C. Nathan Marti, "Development and Predictive Effects of Eating Disorder Risk Factors During Adolescence: Implications for Prevention Efforts," *International Journal of Eating Disorders* 48, no. 2 (2015): 187–98, https://doi.org/10.1002/eat.22270; Eric Stice, C. Nathan Marti, and Shelley Durant, "Risk Factors for Onset of Eating Disorders: Evidence of Multiple Risk Pathways from an 8-Year Prospective Study," *Behaviour Research and Therapy* 49, no. 10 (2011): 622–7, https://doi.org/10.1016/j.brat.2011.06.009; Eric Stice and Heather E. Shaw, "Role of Body Dissatisfaction in the Onset and Maintenance of Eating Pathology: A Synthesis of Research Findings," *Journal of Psychosomatic Research* 53, no. 5 (2002): 985–93, https://doi.org/10.1016/S0022-3999(02)00488-9; Pamela K. Keel, David J. Dorer, Debra L. Franko, Safia C. Jackson, and David B. Herzog, "Postremission Predictors of Relapse in Women with Eating Disorders," *American Journal of Psychiatry* 162, no. 12 (2005), https://doi.org/10.1176/appi.ajp.162.12.2263.

21 Jennifer A. Harriger, Joshua A. Evans, J. Kevin Thompson, and Tracy L. Tylka, "The Dangers of the Rabbit Hole: Reflections on Social Media as a Portal into a Distorted World of Edited Bodies and Eating Disorder Risk and the Role of Algorithms," *Body Image* 41 (2022): 292–7, https://doi.org/10.1016/j.bodyim.2022.03.007; Barbara Jiotsa, Benjamin Naccache, Mélanie Duval, Bruno Rocher, and Marie Grall-Bronnec, "Social Media Use and Body Image Disorders: Association between Frequency of Comparing One's Own Physical Appearance to That of People Being Followed on Social Media and Body Dissatisfaction and Drive for Thinness," *International Journal of Environmental Research and Public Health* 18, no. 6 (2021): 2880, https://doi.org/10.3390/ijerph18062880; Markey, *Adultish: The Body Image Book.*

22 Markey, *Adultish: The Body Image Book.*

23 Phil Reed, Tegan Fowkes, and Mariam Khela, "Reduction in Social Media Usage Produces Improvements in Physical Health and Wellbeing: An RCT," *Journal of Technology in Behavioral Science* 8 (2023): 140–7, https://doi.org/10.1007/s41347-023-00304-7; Olivia E. Smith, Jennifer Mills, and Lindsay Samson, "Out of the Loop: Taking a One-Week Break from Social Media Leads to Better Self-Esteem and Body Image Among Young Women," *Body Image* 49 (2024): 101715, https://doi.org/10.1016/j.bodyim.2024.101715.

24 Charlotte Markey, personal communication, April 27, 2025.

25 Jasmine Fardouly, Amy Slater, Jade Parnell, and Phillippa C. Diedrichs, "Can Following Body Positive or Appearance Neutral Facebook Pages Improve Young Women's Body Image and Mood? Testing Novel Social Media Micro-Interventions," *Body Image* 44 (2023): 136–47, https://doi.org/10.1016/j.bodyim.2022.12.008.

26 You can find EFFT workshops and resources for caregivers at https://mentalhealthfoundations.ca/caregivers and at https://dradelelafrance.com/efft.

27 George T. Doran, "There's a S.M.A.R.T. Way to Write Management's Goals and Objectives," *Management Review* 70, no. 11 (1981): 35, https://community.mis.temple.edu/mis0855002fall2015/files/2015/10/S.M.A.R.T-Way-Management-Review.pdf.

28 Andrria Bianchi, Katherine Stanley, and Kalam Sutandar, "The Ethical Defensibility of Harm Reduction and Eating Disorders," *American Journal of Bioethics* 21, no. 7 (2020): 46–56, https://doi.org/10.1080/15265161.2020.1863509; Edwin Birch, James Downs, and Agnes Ayton, "Harm Reduction in Severe and Long-Standing Anorexia Nervosa: Part of the Journey but Not the Destination—A Narrative Review with Lived Experience," *Journal of Eating Disorders* 12 (2024): 140, https://doi.org/10.1186/s40337-024-01063-3.

29 Laura Kiely, Janet Conti, and Phillipa Hay, "Anorexia Nervosa Through the Lens of a Severe and Enduring Experience: 'Lost in a Big World,'" *Journal of Eating Disorders* 12 (2024): 12, https://doi.org/10.1186/s40337-023-00953-2.

30 Lindsay M. Howard, Anna K. Olson, Brianna N. Pitz, and Kristin E. Heron, "The Role of Denial in Eating Disorder Development, Assessment, and Treatment," in *Eating Disorders*, ed. Vinood Patel and Victor Preedy

(Springer Cham, 2022), 1–17, https://doi.org/10.1007/978-3-030-67929-3_22-1.

31 Christoph Flükiger, A. C. Del Re, Bruce E. Wampold, & Adam O. Horvath, "The Alliance in Adult Psychotherapy: A Meta-Analytic Synthesis," *Psychotherapy* 55, no. 4 (2018): 316–20, https://doi.org/10.1037/pst0000172.

Chapter 7

1 Some quotes that follow were altered slightly (e.g., to fit the format); the heart of the matter did not change.

2 Alli Spotts-De Lazzer, "You're Not Alone, Not the Only One Experiencing this, and People Can Help: Loving Someone with an Eating Disorder," FEAST, published March 4, 2021, https://feast-ed.org/youre-not-alone-not-the-only-one-experiencing-this-and-people-can-help-loving-someone-with-an-eating-disorder/.

3 Carolyn Costin and Alli Spotts-De Lazzer. "To Tell or Not to Tell: Therapists With a Personal History of an Eating Disorder," Eating Disorders Catalogue, published November 30, 2016, https://www.edcatalogue.com/tell-not-tell.

Index

About the Authors

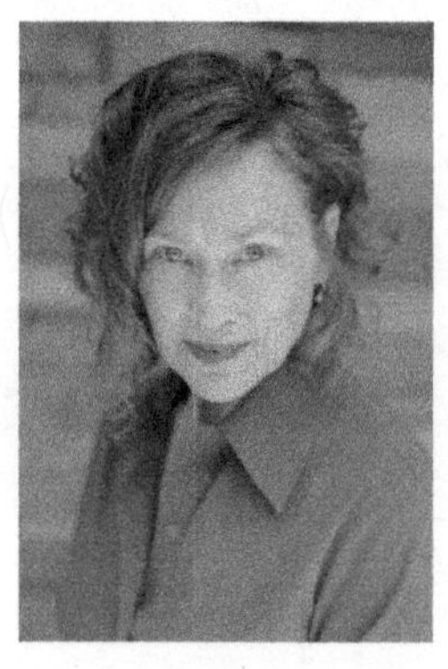

Alli Spotts-De Lazzer is a speaker, author, educator, and psychotherapist. Her credentials include licensed marriage and family therapist (CA 49842 and TN 2657), licensed professional clinical counselor (CA 844), and certified eating disorders specialist (CEDS) with CEDS-approved consultant. Drawing from both professional expertise and personal recovery, Alli offers a uniquely informed and compassionate perspective on eating disorders.

Her public-facing efforts focus on raising awareness about eating and body image issues. Alli authored the book *MeaningFULL: 23 Life-Changing Stories of Conquering Dieting, Weight, & Body Image Issues*, contributed to *Body Image and Self-Esteem*, and created a series of public mental health events—#ShakeIt for Self-Acceptance!—to promote eating disorders awareness nationally through fun and flash mob dance. Since 2021, she has written a *Psychology Today* online column, "MeaningFULL: Candid Perspectives on Self-Image and Mental Health," and since 2011, facilitated a support group for parents and caregivers of individuals with eating disorders.

Alli is deeply committed to contributing to the field of eating disorders. She has published numerous educational articles in academic journals and trade magazines, presented for national eating disorders organizations, lectured at major conferences and universities, designed curricula and taught for the national CEDS, and co-chaired committees for the Academy for Eating Disorders and the International Association of Eating Disorders Professionals (IAEDP).

Honors include being featured as an expert in news outlets that include *The Washington Post* and *The Wall Street Journal*, receiving the IAEDP 2017 Member of the Year award, being an invited expert reviewer for the *American Psychiatric Association Practice Guideline for the Treatment of Patients with Eating Disorders* 2022 draft, and having "#ShakeIt for Self-Acceptance! Day" declared in the City of Los Angeles by Mayor Garcetti. For info: www.therapyhelps.us and www.liveyourfullstory.com

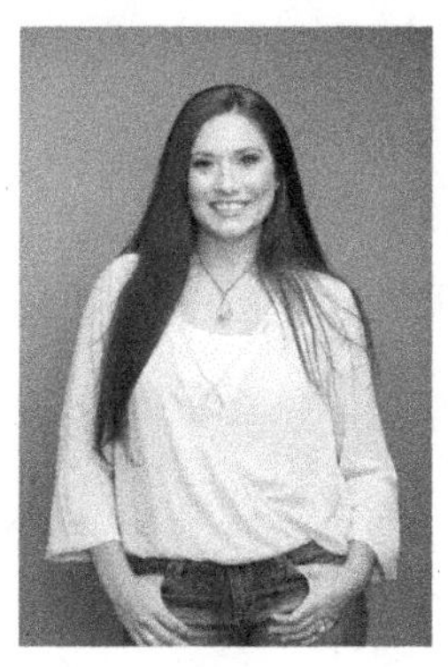

Jenny Mullaney is a certified eating disorder recovery coach (CCIEDC 1010). Since 2017, her certification and coaching practice have been supervised directly by world-renowned eating disorders expert, Carolyn Costin.

Jenny is one of the few recovery coaches worldwide who is hired to live at home with clients during various stages of recovery, serving both as a provider and family advocate. She has thousands of hours of specialized experience in her unique role.

Jenny suffered from her own eating disorder, attending the original Monte Nido Treatment Center in 2005. The philosophy and staff resonated with her so deeply that it ultimately led her to a place of being fully recovered.

Jenny is a contributing writer to Andrea Michal's *Tribe of Light: How Community Helps Us Heal.* Jenny holds a B.A. in liberal studies from Antioch University, is a certified reiki practitioner, and part of The Project HEAL Healer's Circle.

Between recovery coaching travels, she can be found dancing, playing piano, and performing stand-up comedy while residing in Greenwich Village, NY with her eighteen-year-old cat, Seven. For info: www.recoveredispossible.com and https://www.instagram.com/jennymullaney